Understanding
Sleeplessness

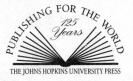
PUBLISHING FOR THE WORLD
125 Years
THE JOHNS HOPKINS UNIVERSITY PRESS

Understanding Sleeplessness

Perspectives on Insomnia

David N. Neubauer, M.D.
Department of Psychiatry and Behavioral Sciences
Johns Hopkins University School of Medicine
Baltimore, Maryland

Foreword by
Paul R. McHugh, M.D.

The Johns Hopkins University Press
Baltimore and London

The Johns Hopkins University Press
2715 North Charles Street
Baltimore, Maryland 21218-4363
www.press.jhu.edu

Library of Congress Cataloging-in-Publication Data

Neubauer, David N., 1951–
  Understanding sleeplessness : perspectives on insomnia / David N.
Neubauer ; foreword by Paul R. McHugh.
      p. ; cm.
Includes bibliographical references and index.
  ISBN 0-8018-7326-6 (hardcover : alk. paper)
  1. Sleep disorders.   I. Title.
  [DNLM: 1. Sleep Initiation and Maintenance Disorders—psychology.   2.
Sleep—physiology. WM 188 N533u 2003]
  RC547 .N485 2003
  616.8'498—dc21
                                                                2002152162

A catalog record for this book is available from the British Library.

Contents

Foreword

A merican psychiatrists are living and practicing in what will someday be called the Checklist Era. In this day and age, the authoritative *Diagnostic and Statistical Manual of Mental Disorders* (DSM) directs us to probe patients for the group A criteria symptoms, group B associated symptoms, and group C exclusionary symptoms of mental illnesses and then to shape our diagnostic opinions and therapeutic plans according to formulae tied to the symptom tally. The Checklist Era has brought us uniformity in diagnosis and improved communication among investigators. But it has also brought automated therapeutics (to be provided in 15-minute time slots, if you please), dubious diagnostic entities, diminished sensitivity to patient suffering, and a collapse of intellectual vitality in psychiatry to a level not seen since the days of physical restraints.

The modern turn in medicine came in the nineteenth century when doctors realized that symptoms and complaints are more than tickets for the sickbed or adequate marks for classification, that they are expressions of underlying life processes, and that the actions of these life processes in the body require systematic study and understanding. Then the complaints manifested by patients could be differentiated and catalogued according to their causes, treated rationally rather than symptomatically, and followed by research linking physicians to the natural sciences surrounding them. Psychiatry has been slow to make this turn—in part because of enthusiasm for its symptomatic treatments—and is now paying a heavy price. Nowhere is this more obvious than with the complaint of insomnia—a complaint possible to dismiss, given the availability of effective pharmacological sedatives, but just as easy to overlook as it slips from attention into the group B thickets of DSM-IV.

With this book, David Neubauer provides a coherent approach to the study of insomnia. (Indeed, he has in the process provided a model for the study of other psychiatric complaints.) Here is a thorough, case-illustrated account of the links tying insomnia to the characteristics of "normal" sleep—

links that give significance to this common complaint and reveal it as a problem to be studied in psychological terms familiar to all psychiatrists.

Dr. Neubauer describes how insomnia can emerge from the homeostatic and circadian features of sleep life: sometimes as a feature of the sleep-wake drive itself, sometimes as an aspect of a patient's unique constitution, sometimes as a response to distressing personal encounters, and sometimes as a feature of a disease of body or brain. In the process, Dr. Neubauer provides not a recipe book for therapeutics (though therapies emerge) nor a catalogue of syndromes (though syndromes are described) but a comprehensive description of how an informed health care provider can skillfully evaluate and treat a common complaint by combining knowledge of basic science and standard explanatory methods. Here is "translational" research (the contemporary term) at its best.

I celebrate this book not only for its achievement but also for what it portends: other monographs and treatises on other psychiatric complaints appreciated and studied, as here, from the "bottom up." This approach springs from information on the manifestations and mechanisms of psychological life as we know it, illuminates the nature of the disruptions to which this life is vulnerable, and delivers an appreciation of psychological symptoms as expressions of life under altered circumstances susceptible to empathic understanding and rational treatment. With this approach we will see the end to the Checklist Era in which patients are "checked out" for complaints in a "top-down" way, with hope that we will stumble upon treatments to manage the complaint.

Think of this book as a prototype of others to come—addressing such complaints as worry, sadness, jealousy, confusion, and the like in exactly the same way. Each of these impending books will reveal an evaluative process, thorough in the office and supplemented by the laboratory, leading to vitality in the doctor-patient relationship, coherent therapeutics, and the encouragement of further research. I predict that they will all repeat what is found thoroughly spelled out here: explicit descriptions of each of the traditional psychiatric explanatory methods—the perspectives of psychiatry, as we came to call them at Johns Hopkins—known since the turn of the twentieth century but rendered invisible during the Checklist Era, to the detriment of our discipline.

Paul R. McHugh, M.D.

Acknowledgments

The plan for this book evolved over several years. I am indebted to many people for their varied contributions to the project.

First, I must thank the patients with whom I have had the opportunity to work at the Sleep Disorders Center at Johns Hopkins. They have taught me about the experiences of having disturbances of sleeping and waking and have stimulated my own continued education and my desire to understand their clinical problems.

I also owe a debt of gratitude to my colleagues in the field of sleep medicine, particularly my associates in the American Academy of Sleep Medicine and the Sleep Research Society. From them I have learned the basics of sleep physiology and clinical sleep medicine.

I am grateful to my mentors in the Department of Psychiatry and Behavioral Sciences at the Johns Hopkins University School of Medicine. Clearly, this book would not have been possible without the teachings of Paul McHugh and Phillip Slavney. I owe them special thanks.

I very much appreciate the collegial relationships and multidisciplinary structure of the Sleep Disorders Center at Johns Hopkins, which have fostered my own development in this clinical specialty. I am particularly grateful to my fellow sleep medicine faculty members Philip Smith, Alan Schwartz, Naresh Punjabi, Seva Polotsky, Nancy Collop, Christopher Earley, Richard Allen, and Suzanne Lesage for stimulating discussions and debates.

Several individuals read selected chapters or the entire manuscript as I was writing this book. I am grateful to all of them for helpful suggestions. Among them are Paul McHugh, Phillip Slavney, David Edwin, Michael Smith, and Kristin Mears.

I have had the opportunity to speak with many groups of physicians and other health care professionals about sleep disorders in general and insomnia in particular. These valuable discussions have helped me understand the many ways in which sleep problems are viewed and the challenges of addressing them in clinical practice.

I appreciate the encouragement and valuable help throughout the development of this project from the Johns Hopkins University Press, especially that of my editors, Wendy Harris and Linda Forlifer.

Finally, I must thank my parents, Richard and Winnie Neubauer, for encouragement and support throughout my education, and my immediate family, Lynne, Rebecca, and Robert, for their understanding while I have been hidden away with my laptop, writing this book.

Understanding
Sleeplessness

1

The Problems with Insomnia

Insomnia has many consequences, yet it is difficult to diagnose precisely.

Insomnia is a common problem in our society, and it represents a major clinical challenge. Sleeplessness is one of the most frequent complaints people present to their physicians. Millions of Americans suffer with it, and billions of dollars are spent annually trying to treat it. The consequences of insomnia are quite varied and include the obvious individual suffering and huge societal costs. In spite of the magnitude of this problem, there is considerable debate in the health care establishment about what insomnia is and what should be done about it.

The causes of insomnia have been the focus of many research studies. These have explored sleep complaints in association with epidemiology, psychological and neurophysiological correlates, medical and psychiatric disorders, and assorted treatment strategies. Research has been done primarily with humans but also with animal models. With increasing scientific knowledge of both the psychological and the physiological characteristics of normal sleep, it is more evident that a multitude of factors can undermine the experience of good sleep (Gillin and Byerley, 1990). Sleep specialists concur that the etiology of insomnia usually is multifactorial. Even when a single cause of sleeplessness seems obvious, other processes usually contribute to the problem in persistent cases.

Varied potential causes and a myriad of solutions have filled articles and books in the popular press. Some present current evidence-based treatment recommendations and serve an important function in helping to educate a wide audience. Some lack sound scientific support but have reasonable foundations and offer harmless and possibly helpful advice.

Others are patently misguided and join that genre of health literature that seduces the sufferer away from appropriate and effective help.

The scientific literature on insomnia reflects the significant diversity of conceptual models used in hypotheses attempting to explain insomnia. The more popular writings expand this range of explanatory approaches even further. The purpose of this book is to explore the conceptual models that support different understandings of what insomnia is and what should be done about it. The goal here is not to reveal a single answer but rather to show strengths and weaknesses in the theoretical models. Ultimately, this enterprise should promote a broad approach in evaluating and treating individuals with insomnia. With a broad approach, critical factors potentially influencing the sleep-wake cycle can be highlighted.

This chapter reviews the ambiguity of the term *insomnia*, the epidemiology of insomnia complaints, the consequences of this sleep disturbance, the primary treatment strategies, and the limitations of medical education on normal sleep and sleep disorders. I explain the functions of sleep disorders centers and discuss the four perspectives as explanatory models.

What Is Insomnia?

The word *insomnia* is derived from the Latin *somnus* (sleep) and thus suggests the state of not being in sleep. The term is used in many ways in our vernacular language as well as in medical and scientific literature but always with a negative connotation. Although most people agree about the general meaning of the word, it is ambiguous in not specifying a particular pattern of sleep difficulty or underlying problem. Fundamentally, "I have insomnia" means (1) "I can't sleep" and (2) "I'm suffering." There are many variations on insomnia-related complaints:

- It takes me too long to fall asleep at night.
- I keep waking up throughout the night; it seems like every hour.
- I never get deep sleep anymore; I'm always in a twilight state.
- I haven't slept in months.
- I always wake up too early and can't get back to sleep.
- My mind just won't shut off at night.
- I always have to drag myself out of bed in the morning because my nighttime sleep is so bad.

- I never feel rested.
- I'm fatigued all day.
- I couldn't nap if my life depended on it.

The first six items relate to the general sense of very light sleep and the specific complaints of difficulty initiating and maintaining sleep. Associated with the usual nighttime problems are daytime symptoms (like the last four items), typically offered as results of the previous night's sleeplessness. Daytime complaints range from fatigue, sleepiness, and inadvertent episodes of sleep to a sense of excessive arousal and a complete inability to nap. Of course, this nighttime/daytime discussion assumes a "normal" desired sleep-wake schedule, which increasingly is made difficult by current lifestyles. Accordingly, the insomnia complaint may come from the shift worker unable to sleep when the opportunity is available during daylight hours and having difficulty functioning effectively on the nighttime work shift. In contemporary society the general definition of insomnia can be expanded to "I'm suffering because I can't sleep *when I want to sleep*." (Throughout this book, it will be assumed that nighttime is the desired sleep time, unless otherwise indicated.)

Although daytime problems are an important component of the overall insomnia complaint, these symptoms alone do not constitute evidence of insomnia. There must always be a direct experience of insufficient sleep, not simply the supposition that sleep is impaired because one feels unrefreshed in the morning or throughout the day. Many processes can promote daytime fatigue or sleepiness without one having a sense of impaired nighttime sleep. Schedule-induced sleep deprivation, sleep-disordered breathing, and narcolepsy may impair daytime functioning without necessarily also causing an experience of disrupted nighttime sleep. The word *insomnia* is already vague when it refers to inadequate sleep. Attempts to expand the scope of the definition risk dilution of the concept and further confusion about symptoms and causes. An excessively broad definition trivializes the suffering of severely afflicted individuals.

Because the term *insomnia* is so general, further description is necessary to characterize an individual's complaint. Quite important is the timing of the sleep disturbance. Is there a predominant pattern of difficulty falling asleep, frequent or prolonged awakenings, early-morning arousals without return to sleep, or a combination of these? The severity can range from mild to extreme, and the complaint may include the minutes and hours of sleep achieved or lost. The duration may range from acute (a few days) to chronic (insomnia of weeks, months, or years). Frequency may be nightly or intermittent with a predictable or seemingly random pattern. A weekly, monthly, or seasonal sleep disturbance may be evident, or there may be a regular association with recurrent life events. Similarly, the daytime symptoms of fatigue, sleepiness, or excessive arousal may be characterized by severity, time of day, and effect on daytime functioning.

The subjective nature of the insomnia complaint makes it difficult to apply objective criteria to define the sleep problem. One might try to circumscribe insomnia formally in terms of numbers. For instance, a patient could meet a particular insomnia criterion by taking more than x minutes to fall asleep y nights per week for z weeks. Alternatively, a patient could awaken x times per night with a total wake period of y minutes and no more than z hours of sleep for the night. One could develop similar criteria to define early-morning awakening. Such a rigid and objective approach is of little value in the clinical realm. It is the *experience* of insufficient sleep that creates the insomniac, not the actual minutes or hours without sleep. Nevertheless, researchers must use some criteria to categorize individuals for epidemiological studies or clinical therapeutic trials. Surveyors may classify groups by numbers (e.g., minutes awake, nights per week), but these still usually represent subjective reports of sleeplessness.

There is a surprisingly weak correspondence between subjective reports by insomnia complainers and objective measurements of their sleep parameters. Sleep laboratory investigations suggest that the subjective sleep estimates of insomniacs often exaggerate the difficulty initiating and maintaining sleep in comparison with the objective electroencephalogram (EEG) sleep standards (Carskadon et al., 1976). Many people complaining of insomnia clearly misperceive their actual sleep. Recruitment of insomniac persons for research projects is rather challenging, as many insomnia responders sleep too well in the laboratory on screening nights to be included in an insomnia group defined by objective criteria. This limited correlation between the subjective sleep report and the objective laboratory sleep measurement does not suggest that the insomnia problem is not real. Rather, it challenges our understanding of the experience of sleep and waking for these individuals.

The problem of subjective versus objective sleep experience is complicated by the wide variation of sleep characteristics in the general population. Some individuals seem to have average nightly sleep requirements that are particularly long or short, although many people in our society would benefit from more sleep than they allow themselves. There must be a relative influence of the need for sleep on the sleep achieved. One person may sleep six hours, believe that the sleep has been sound, and feel refreshed on awakening in the morning; another may sleep six hours, perceive the sleep as very light and interrupted, and subsequently feel unrefreshed during the daytime.

How long it should take to fall asleep at bedtime is a relevant question without an adequate answer. One person may claim to fall asleep before her head hits the pillow. Another may estimate 40 minutes without complaining. Yet another may describe the agonizing 20 minutes it takes him to fall asleep. Thirty minutes frequently has been offered as a minimum sleep latency (time it takes to fall asleep) to define sleep-onset insomnia. Although this may be a useful value where values are necessary, it must be recognized that insomnia complainers and noncomplainers will fall on both sides of the 30-minute boundary. This is also true with similar criteria for nighttime awakenings and estimates of total sleep time.

Why are some people insomniac and others not so? The first requirements are the perceptions that a lack of sleep exists and that it is a problem. A mental threshold may be crossed regarding the severity of the nighttime sleeplessness or the daytime effects. This conclusion flows from a comparison with what one regards as normal or good sleep. There must be a *sleep expectation,* presumably culturally influenced, against which people measure their current *sleep experience.* Our own cultural ideal seems to be for a rapid onset and then eight hours of uninterrupted sleep that allows one to feel refreshed the following day. For many insomniac persons, it is the daytime effects that eventually bring them in for treatment. Future research may help us better understand the processes influencing the perceptions of individuals complaining of insomnia who objectively demonstrate good sleep according to current sleep laboratory standards.

If the perception of poor sleep makes the person insomniac, what then makes the insomniac person a patient? What influences the insomniac person to seek help from a health care provider for this identified problem? Surveys coordinated by the National Sleep Foundation suggest that a minority of insomnia sufferers come to their health care providers specifically for their sleep problem (Ancoli-Israel and Roth, 1999). Those seen for insomnia in clinical settings represent the tip of the iceberg. Others may not seek help because:

- they believe nothing can be done about the problem
- they are pursuing alternative or "natural" solutions
- they are afraid their physician will view their problem as trivial
- they worry that they will be given a "sleeping pill" that will cause new problems

Perhaps increased public education and enlightened media attention will stimulate greater recognition of sleep disturbance and appropriate treatments and encourage more people to seek help for their sleep-wake problems. Many myths and misconceptions regarding sleep need correction.

Insomnia and Published Nosologies

If we accept that insomnia is a perception-based complaint with a multitude of causes, comorbidities, and reinforcements shifting dynamically through time, then the goal of creating a neat scheme of discrete diagnostic entities becomes unattainable. However, complete diagnostic nihilism is not a satisfactory alternative. Diagnostic classifications are necessary and potentially valuable, however imperfect. Nosologies can maximize the identification and understanding of various factors that may promote and sustain insomnia, but they tend to minimize the notion of multiple simultaneous processes influencing the perception of sleep disturbance. The different approaches to the classification of insomnia are evident in the *Diagnostic and Statistical Manual of Mental Disorders* (4th edition) (DSM-IV) (American Psychiatric Association, 1994), the *International Classification of Diseases* (ICD-9-CM) (American Medical Association, 1996), and the *International Classification of Sleep Disorders: Diagnostic and Coding Manual* (ICSD) (Diagnostic Classification Steering Committee, 1990). In these large-scale nosologies, some definitions of sleep disorders are relatively discrete (e.g., narcolepsy and obstructive sleep apnea); however, insomnia remains somewhat nebulous.

The DSM-IV separates primary sleep disorders from those thought to be related to a mental disorder, a general medical condition, or the effect of a substance (stimulating or sedating). Insomnia may exist in all four of these general categories. The primary sleep disorders subsume the parasomnias (e.g., nightmares, sleep terrors, and sleepwalking) and the dyssomnias, which relate to disturbances in the amount, timing, and quality of sleep. These dyssomnias include primary insomnia, primary hypersomnia, narcolepsy, breathing-related sleep disorder, and circadian rhythm sleep disorder.

According to the DSM-IV, primary insomnia is the complaint of difficulty initiating or maintaining sleep or of nonrestorative sleep lasting one month or longer. Nonrestorative sleep is described as the feeling of restless, light, or poor-quality sleep. Also required is clinically significant distress or impairment associated with the insomnia complaint. Finally, the insomnia must not be attributed to another primary sleep disorder, mental disorder, general medical condition, or effect of a substance. The DSM-IV discussion of features and disorders associated with primary insomnia foreshadows the inherent problems of the nosology boundaries. Primary insomnia may be associated with symptoms of depression and anxiety, but too much of these symptoms may shift the diagnosis to another general category. Complicating this is the recognition that persistent insomnia increases the risk for the development of a new onset of or the recurrence of anxiety or mood disorders (Ford and Kamerow, 1989). If the insomnia came first, should this require a category shift? Can causation and comorbidity be distinguished satisfactorily? A similar problem exists with the substance issue: persistent insomnia symptoms may promote the use of various stimulating or sedating substances (legal or illegal), which in turn leads to a diagnosis of substance abuse or dependence and to the risk of another insomnia category challenge.

Studies have demonstrated moderate inter-rater reliability in the DSM-IV classification system for insomnia; however, this does not establish the degree of validity of these diagnostic categories. Assorted processes can promote insomnia in individuals with all disorders, whether or not a mental disorder is diagnosed. The evaluation of any person complaining of insomnia who also has a diagnosis of a mental disorder may be complicated by an awkward differential diagnosis. Without supporting criteria, evaluators must decide whether they think that the underlying mental disorder (e.g., major depression) is causing the insomnia symptoms or whether the sleep disturbance is independent. If the insomnia is judged to be integral to the mental disorder, then it must be decided whether the insomnia severity is sufficient to warrant the additional diagnosis. The problem is complicated when insomnia is present and a new onset of a mental disorder is considered.

The inherent weaknesses of the DSM-IV are due to the complexity of the evolution and clinical presentation of insomnia symptoms as well as to current limitations in sleep medicine. On the positive side, DSM-IV does highlight certain clinical categories of sleep disturbance that otherwise might not be identified or formally diagnosed.

The ICD-9-CM offers a basic dichotomy of sleep disturbances of presumed organic and nonorganic etiology. Among the nonorganic categories (codes 307.4x) are the transient and persistent disorders of initiating or maintaining sleep. The transient category is associated with emotional reactions or conflicts, and the persistent disorders relate to anxiety, depression, psychosis, and conditioned arousal. Other nonorganic choices include a phase-shift disruption of the 24-hour sleep-wake cycle (e.g., jet lag and shift work) and repetitive intrusions by environmental disturbances or sleep stage abnormalities. A "nonorganic, other" option allows coding for the natural short sleeper and the subjective insomnia complaint. A separate ICD sleep disturbance diagnosis series (codes 780.5x) excludes the above categories of nonorganic origin and thereby assumes organic pathology. Available here are an insomnia NOS (not otherwise specified) option, an unspecified sleep disturbance, dysfunctions associated with sleep stages or arousal from sleep, disruptions of the 24-hour sleep-wake cycle, and insomnia with sleep apnea.

Several problems emerge immediately with the ICD scheme. Although the basic separation into organic and nonorganic causes is appealing conceptually, evidence justifying the distinction is lacking, and arguably it is false in several of the applications. The diagnostic placement of severe but uncomplicated insomnia as organic or nonorganic seems to be at the whim of the coder. Generally, the insomnia entities and the distinctions among them are not well defined. The ICD system is intended for worldwide use, and in many situations ICD coding is mandatory. While ICD classifications may be valid in other medical areas, the insomnia organization does not represent a consensus understanding of this sleep difficulty, nor does it promote consistent diagnosis or treatment. This is especially unfortunate considering the overall influence of the ICD.

Several international professional sleep societies used a process of expert consensus to develop the ICSD diagnostic categories, which have a pathophysiological organization. The process was intended to be multidisciplinary, representing the broad-based interests of several medical specialties involved in sleep medicine. The ICSD system has 3 major categories, with 11 additional diagnostic entities lumped into a proposed sleep disorder group. The general category of dyssomnias relates to disorders resulting in complaints of insomnia or excessive sleepiness. It is divided into subsets of intrinsic sleep disorders, extrinsic sleep disorders, and circadian rhythm sleep disorders. Together these allow for 34 possible diagnoses, of which many may result in an insomnia complaint. The intrinsic sleep disorders are those that arise within the body and primarily cause a sleep disturbance. Among the 13 disorders under this heading are psychophysiological insomnia, idiopathic insomnia, sleep state misperception, narcolepsy, obstructive sleep apnea syndrome, and restless legs syndrome. The extrinsic category incorporates those processes originating or developing from causes outside the body. This suggests that resolution of the external problem, if possible, will improve the associated sleep disturbance. Among the 14 categories are inadequate sleep hygiene, adjustment sleep disorder, insufficient sleep syndrome, and alcohol-dependent sleep disorder. The circadian rhythm disorders relate to the timing of the sleep period as influenced by the internal circadian clock. Examples here include time zone change syndrome, shift work sleep disorder, delayed sleep phase syndrome, and advanced sleep phase syndrome.

Parasomnias are the second major ICSD category. The idea here is that the entities are not primary sleeping and waking problems but rather disorders related to arousal and sleep stage transition. They intrude into or emanate from sleep. The parasomnias are divided into arousal disorders, sleep-wake transition disorders, rapid eye movement (REM) sleep parasomnias, and other parasomnias. Several of these may be related indirectly to the complaint of insomnia. Among the parasomnias are bruxism, sleep terrors, nightmares, sleep paralysis, REM sleep behavior disorder, and sleep enuresis.

The third general ICSD category is sleep disorders associated with medical or psychiatric disorders, and it includes many potential secondary causes of the insomnia complaint. The general category is broken down into the disturbances associated with mental disorders (e.g., psychoses, mood disorders, and anxiety disorders), neurological disorders (e.g., dementia, parkinsonism, and sleep-related epilepsy), and, finally, other medical disorders (e.g., chronic obstructive pulmonary disease, sleep-related asthma, sleep-related gastroesophageal reflux, and various causes of chronic pain).

A major strength of the ICSD is that it elaborates a variety of different processes that can lead to insomnia complaints. The insomnia-related disorders range from those that are measurable physiologically to those based on theoretical constructs and presumed but not readily measurable pathophysiology. The ICSD categories are not entirely discrete, and individual patients with insomnia may be diagnosable in several of the disorder categories. The growing clinical knowledge of sleep disorders has allowed the development of the relatively sophisticated ICSD structure, but current knowledge limitations also limit the construction of a fully adequate outline of insomnia diagnoses. Debate continues over the definitions and applications of the key ICSD insomnia categories. A complete revision of the ICSD nosology now is under way.

Overall, these three nosologies are limited in helping us understand the development and progression of insomnia symptoms or appreciate the dynamic complexity of simultaneous influences. Questions of validity, inter-rater reliability, diagnosis boundary, and symptom inclusion threshold are evident with each of the three insomnia organizations. The ideal insomnia nosology (presently unattainable) would resolve these issues with valid and reliable constructs consistent with current practice and beliefs. It would be useful clinically in helping to direct patient management and would provide a good educational foundation. Finally, it would incorporate a multidimensional structure to emphasize the confluence of processes contributing to an individual's clinical situation.

The Basic Epidemiology of Insomnia

The prevalence of insomnia has been assessed through numerous studies ranging from questionnaires and telephone surveys asking general questions to structured interviews with stringent criteria. The general questions, such as whether one sometimes has trouble sleeping, elicit a relatively high percentage of positive responses. Surveys often suggest that about one-third to one-half of the adult populations of the United States and other Western nations at least occasionally have had insomnia symptoms within the previous year (Ancoli-Israel and Roth, 1999). In contrast, results from surveys and interviews that assess the frequency, chronicity, or perceived severity of insomnia generally include 10-15 percent of these populations as having a serious problem with this sleep disturbance (Zorick and Walsh,

2000). Unfortunately, cross-cultural epidemiological or phenomenological studies of sleep disturbances are practically nonexistent.

Typically, elderly people are at greater risk for insomnia, as are women, particularly beginning with menopause (Owens and Matthews, 1998). Individuals with psychiatric and other medical problems also are at increased risk. As the prevalence of these disorders is greater for older individuals, these disorders account for some of the increase in insomnia associated with aging. Generally, people in medical settings tend to have a higher prevalence of insomnia (Katz and McHorney, 1998). Lower socioeconomic status may be an independent factor associated with increased insomnia (Bixler et al., 1979). The breadth of the insomnia problem is evident in data on health care utilization, including visits to a medical provider, and the use of prescription and over-the-counter (OTC) preparations.

One caveat of the results of large-scale surveys on insomnia is the question of sleep dissatisfaction. When a person complains to a health care provider about poor sleep, the dissatisfaction is evident. However, one can respond positively to insomnia criteria on a survey without being significantly dissatisfied with sleep and without regarding the sleep characteristic as a clinical problem. Extrapolating large percentages estimated from surveys to indicate the societal burden of insomnia risks considerable exaggeration.

The Consequences of Insomnia

By definition, insomnia involves the experience of inadequate nighttime sleep. During the night there is a sense of wakefulness and possibly distress about the inability to sleep soundly. The potential daytime consequences are quite varied, with acute and chronic effects. A general tendency is for acute insomnia to result in daytime sleepiness but for chronic insomnia to be associated with daytime arousal. Overall, persistent insomnia can have significant and serious consequences for public health, quality of life, and economics. There also may be physiological effects from associated sleep deprivation.

Several studies have examined particular outcome measures in defined insomnia populations and matched controls (Johnson and Spinweber, 1983; Zammit et al., 1999). Typically, the insomnia subjects are more likely to report symptoms of depression, irritability, fatigue, decreased concentration, and memory difficulty. They feel less productive at work and report more missed days. There may be less occupational advancement. Some studies suggest that persons with insomnia have more driving accidents.

Quality-of-life issues are pronounced among people who complain of insomnia. Standardized rating scales, including instruments specifically measuring quality of life (SF-36, QOL Inventory), show statistically significant reductions in function and increases in self-perceived health problems in the insomnia populations. The recognition of this correlation is important; however, the relative strength of the causation directions is not established. Some degree of circularity and perpetuation would be expected.

Depressive symptoms often are associated with the presence of insomnia. Clearly, depressive disorders almost always cause insomnia. However, insomnia also may cause the symptoms of depression and increase the risk of new-onset major depression. Retrospective and prospective studies of large-scale and well-defined focused populations support this conclusion (Ford and Kamerow, 1989; Breslau et al., 1996; Chang et al., 1997). The presence of insomnia in baseline and follow-up surveys predicts the development of major depression. The question remains whether the initial insomnia simply increases the risk of the depressive disorder or whether the insomnia is a prodromal symptom, the first sign of depression to come. Nevertheless, these findings emphasize the importance of early recognition and treatment of insomnia.

People with insomnia, whether or not it is an identified clinical problem, tend to have greater overall health care costs (Walsh and Engelhardt, 1999; Simon and VonKorff, 1997). The increased costs may, in part, be due to the expense of working up insomnia-related symptoms (e.g., fatigue and tiredness) and to medications prescribed to treat underlying disorders and promote a direct hypnotic effect. They also likely reflect the increased risk of insomnia in people with other medical disorders (Katz and McHorney, 1998).

Researchers have extrapolated large-scale societal costs based on population estimates and presumed consequences of insomnia (Stoller, 1994). Reasonably conservative projections of direct costs typically are in the range of several billions of dollars annually, and the expense of just the prescription and OTC substances taken to treat insomnia in the United States is more than one billion dollars each year. The addition of indirect and related costs of insomnia would amplify these values tremendously. It is evident that this multitude of costs and consequences of insomnia produces a huge economic burden in our society.

General Approaches to Treatment

The responses to insomnia vary enormously. Of course, the severity, duration, and presumed cause of the sleep disturbance influence what, if anything, one might do in the attempt to improve sleep. Many people do nothing purposeful to solve the insomnia and hope that their sleep will improve spontaneously. Some people turn to folk remedies or other solutions that they believe will be beneficial (e.g., a glass of wine at bedtime) but that turn out to cause greater sleep disturbance. Others try going to bed earlier or staying up later to get more sleep or fall asleep more quickly. Many people try the familiar advice for good sleep hygiene: avoid caffeine; sleep in a quiet, dark, and cool room; avoid bed except for sleep and sex; and resist daytime napping.

Some people with insomnia may be motivated to participate in behavioral programs involving sleep logs, schedule changes, and more time out of bed (Bootzin and Perlis, 1992). They may be treated psychotherapeutically to deal with underlying conflicts or to reframe cognitive distortions about their sleep (Morin et al., 1999; Edinger et al., 2001). Desperation leads people to try various medicinal approaches, which may include vitamins and herbal remedies. Preparations of untested effectiveness and safety that are promoted as sleep aids fill store shelves. People try OTC antihistamines, take leftover prescription medications from family and friends, and, finally, sometimes obtain medications from their physicians.

Health care providers may recommend assorted medications with the goal of improving sleep. Of course, some medications are directed at associated psychiatric and other medical disorders that may be contributing to the insomnia. Prescribed medications given with the primary intention of a hypnotic effect include higher-dose antihistamines, barbiturates and related compounds (fortunately rare now), some antidepressants, and benzodiazepine receptor agonists. Usage varies among physicians and patients. Generally, the hypnotics are recommended for short-term use (days to weeks); however, some people take them most nights for months to years.

Most people who would respond positively on a survey of insomnia symptoms do not seek professional help for the problem; still, there are plenty who do request help. How a patient complaining of poor sleep is evaluated and managed by a physician or other health care professional depends greatly on that provider's training, experience, knowledge, and attitudes. Practices vary widely with regard to history taking, patient education, behavioral approaches, and the use of different types of medications. Overlapping and loosely defined diagnostic labels for insomnia are used. Clearly, this situation does not enhance the identification, evaluation, or treatment of patients.

Education in Sleep Medicine

Some degree of blame for the health care establishment's deficiencies in adequately identifying and treating insomnia patients rests with traditions in medical education. Generally, sleep and sleep disorders have been ignored in medical and other health care training programs (Rosen et al., 1993). Many medical schools have no training regarding sleep whatsoever, and very few provide more than a few hours of attention. Multiple factors have contributed to this relative neglect of sleep-related topics. The basic science and clinical issues concerning sleep cross many academic departmental boundaries, and no single established field has evolved a national mandate to promote general education in sleep medicine. The recognition of the importance to health of sleep habits and sleep disorders, as well as of the foundations of normal and abnormal sleep in basic science, has emerged rapidly and comparatively recently. There has been resistance to the incorporation of new topics into medical school curricula, which already are highly competitive for time and resources. Other recognized barriers include a shortage of trained faculty, a lack of interdisciplinary programming on sleep, and limited recognition of the relative importance of sleep medicine. Major changes in health care education will be necessary locally and nationally as a comprehensive sleep medicine curriculum is developed and implemented in training programs, as well as in continuing education programs for practicing physicians.

Sleep Disorders Centers

Patients seek help in sleep disorders centers, independently or referred by their physicians, for problems ranging from insomnia to excessive sleepiness to the assorted abnormal behaviors and other symptoms (parasomnias) that occur in relation to their sleep. Insomnia is by far the most common sleep complaint in the general population, but excessive sleepiness motivates a large proportion of affected individuals to pursue evaluation at a sleep disorders center. This is because of the detrimental effects of excessive sleepiness, including occupational impairment (e.g., falling asleep at the keyboard) and safety concerns (e.g., falling asleep at the wheel). Recent media attention to the dangers of excessive sleepiness and the health problems associated with sleep-disordered breathing certainly contributes to these referrals. Overall, referrals to sleep disorders centers have increased dramatically over the past two decades. A recent survey of 19 U.S. sleep centers totaling more than four thousand patients showed that two-thirds ultimately were diagnosed with sleep-disordered breathing (Punjabi, Welch, and Strohl, 2000). Only 5 percent received a primary ICSD diagnosis of an insomnia disorder, although about 15 percent offered insomnia as a presenting symptom.

Sleep disorders centers in the United States may be accredited by the American Academy of Sleep Medicine, and currently there are more than five hundred member centers. Accreditation criteria include the participation of a board-certified (American Board of Sleep Medicine) physician or psychologist at the sleep center. Accordingly, the center is expected to be able to evaluate and treat patients with the full spectrum of sleep disorders. In contrast, many recently opened sleep centers focus solely on diagnostic testing for sleep-disordered breathing.

The initial evaluation in a sleep center typically involves a comprehensive history, including a detailed review of issues relevant to the sleep-wake cycle and symptoms of particular sleep disorders, and a physical examination. If indicated, the person may be referred for sleep laboratory testing. This polysomnographic testing is common for patients with excessive daytime sleepiness; however, not all insomnia patients will require laboratory testing. Generally, it is reserved for those cases where it is suspected that another primary sleep disorder may be contributing to the insomnia symptoms.

The Johns Hopkins Sleep Disorders Center has evolved over the past three decades into an active clinical and research facility. The associated sleep laboratory has six beds available for sleep studies. This sleep disorders center is multidisciplinary, with faculty from the departments of pulmonary medicine, neurology, and psychiatry. About one thousand new patients are evaluated annually.

Throughout this book, clinical vignettes drawn mostly from my now

18-year experience on the faculty at the Johns Hopkins Sleep Disorders Center illustrate different patient presentations related to the complaint of insomnia. (The patient names have been changed to protect confidentiality.) The brief histories offer the salient features but not necessarily all of the negative findings in the cases. Many of the examples are typical of the insomnia patients commonly evaluated and treated by psychiatrists, primary care physicians, and other health care providers. It should be evident that widely divergent processes can result in similar presentations, just as patients may manifest similar underlying processes in very different ways. As in all of medicine, a thorough history is vital and should lead to a useful differential diagnosis and treatment plan.

The Four Perspectives

In considering the conceptual models used to explain insomnia, this book draws heavily on the approach elaborated in *The Perspectives of Psychiatry*, by Paul McHugh and Phillip Slavney (second edition, 1998). These authors explore fundamental explanatory models, and their relation to diagnosis and treatment, in the field of psychiatry. Different disciplines and orientations within the field are viewed as having complementary partial understandings, each illuminating aspects of psychopathology with unique strengths and inherent limitations. McHugh and Slavney argue that psychiatric reasoning can be approached from four major perspectives: the disease model, the dimensional approach, the motivated behavior paradigm, and the life-story method. Clinical situations are most valuably formulated by using several perspectives simultaneously. The recognition that these perspectives are not mutually exclusive helps prevent the parochialism that has plagued the field of psychiatry in the past. The result is greater integration in understanding and care of patients.

The disease perspective is category driven in the attempt to create patient clusters. The ultimate goal is the definition of discrete diseases based on identifiable pathological conditions. The dimensional perspective considers variation and gradation. Individual vulnerability is emphasized in relation to one's position along gradations of human variation. The behavioral perspective recognizes several goal-directed behaviors fundamental and necessary to human existence. For instance, drives related to sleeping, eating, and sexual behaviors can be posited and then described as normal or abnormal. The life-story perspective is based on a narrative logic that makes one's response to circumstances empathically understandable.

The potential benefit of applying the perspectives approach to the problem of insomnia is evident. Each of these approaches offers valuable and complementary insights into the assessment of the individual with insomnia complaints and therefore can enhance our understanding of the many influences on the experience of sleep. Like many aspects of psychopathology, symptoms of insomnia are complex and poorly quantifiable, not easily ordered into specifically labeled states. Just as there is probably not a single disease of schizophrenia, there is not a single insomnia.

Throughout this book it should be evident that influences emphasized by the four conceptual models may contribute to the vulnerability for insomnia, precipitate acute sleep problems, or help sustain chronic symptoms. Chapter 2 offers a broad overview of normal sleep with which to contrast the pathology of insomnia. Most of this book consists of chapters devoted to each of the four perspectives and to how our understanding of the evolution, phenomenology, and treatment of insomnia is elucidated by that point of view. The book concludes with a chapter recommending an integrative approach that takes advantage of the strengths of the disease, dimensional, motivated behavior, and life-story perspectives. A comprehensive evaluation of a patient complaining of insomnia will have considered the influences inherent in all of these realms of explanation and will result in a formulation and treatment plan addressing all of the relevant issues.

Summary

Insomnia fundamentally is a perception and an interpretation. Whether the complaint is supported objectively is a separate issue, although relevant and interesting in any particular case. Generally, insomnia is multifactorial in etiology and should be understood in many ways simultaneously. This does not necessarily mean several concomitant disease states but, rather, a confluence of processes and factors related to personal vulnerability, situational stresses, sleepiness drive, and the individual's intrinsic and extrinsic environments. There is no simple unifying conceptual theory for insomnia that will generate a single answer. However, appreciating the complexity of the elements initiating and perpetuating the experience of sleep disturbance certainly will allow better direction of treatment and improvement in outcomes. Fortunately, the recognition of a complex etiological field does not necessarily translate to hopelessly complicated patient management. A broad vision of sleep experience enhances the recognition of the critical problems to be addressed. Furthermore, one treatment strategy may have therapeutic implications across perspective boundaries. This may involve sleep-wake schedule reorganization, the underlying sleepiness drive, a decreased sense of futility, and a reduced anxiety state.

Insomnia is a common concern with considerable individual and societal consequences. Effective recognition and management has great potential benefit in improved quality of life, reduced morbidity, and decreased economic burden. This can be achieved only with an appreciation of the potential interrelations of factors together influencing sleep and wakefulness.

2

Normal Sleep

What We Know and How We Know It

Insomnia can exist only with reference to what one believes is normal sleep.

What Is Normal?

Insomnia is a subjective complaint. The reason one experiences insomnia may be simple and obvious, or it may be complex, multifactorial, and elusive. In all cases, however, people conclude that they have insomnia by comparing their sleep and wakefulness with their personal expectations of normal sleep and subsequent alertness. The central question is, "What is normal sleep?" This question raises several challenging and not fully resolvable issues.

The initial problem is that the characteristics of expected normal sleep are relative. Different people will draw varying conclusions about when their sleep experience deviates significantly from a presumed norm. Consequences, especially the sense of suffering during the nighttime and daytime, as well as any other perceived impairment, affect when a person will complain of insomnia.

The next major difficulty in the attempt explicitly to define normal sleep is the source of the standard. For instance, normal sleep may be viewed as synonymous with ideal sleep, such that anything less than the imagined perfect sleep is insomnia. Alternatively, normal sleep may be interpreted as typical sleep (i.e., normal being the general sleep characteristics of one's peers). From this viewpoint, normal sleep can be approached by assessing the sleep of various populations, such as groupings according to age and sex. Attention to the cultural context should help maximize the validity of the standard. Survey data can offer a representation of how most people in a population think that they typically sleep. Longitudinal assessments with sleep logs can present a more accurate reflection of sleep characteristics within a sample. Finally, physiological monitoring can be used to address the question of normality of sleep for individuals by comparing various parameters, such as the electroencephalogram (EEG), with accepted scientific standards. Scientific criteria are necessary, valuable, and the product of extensive and creative investigation, but they still signify only a consensus state-of-the-art definition at any particular time. Accordingly, new technology, discovery, and theoretical development undoubtedly will bring changes in the understanding of the essential features embodying what is considered normal sleep. Even then, the ultimate physiological standards of normality may not ever correspond completely with the subjective experiences of sleep or sleeplessness. Consider the importance of how the following patient interprets his sleep experience and eventually decides that he suffers from insomnia.

Thomas was a 37-year-old single business executive when he requested a consultation regarding his longstanding sleep problems. He described a sense of having experienced light and disrupted sleep for several years. Asked when it started, he responded that he did not know. He was able, however, to offer the month five years previously when he had realized that he suffered from insomnia. He said that somehow he had experienced a great night of sleep and more energy the following day, and he concluded that something had been wrong with his sleep, since it was not like that all of the time. After that single satisfying night, he returned to the nighttime sleep disruption and daytime fatigue. He sought help from several physicians and tried a variety of medications, including antidepressants and hypnotics. These medications had been of limited value in providing him with a sense of normal sleep and daytime alertness.

This book emphasizes how the complaint of insomnia may be conceptualized and explained and how these explanatory models influence what the individual sufferers and those around them, including their health care providers, do about the problem. The objective of this chapter is to review the broad understandings of sleep that have evolved from scientific investigations over the past several decades, including the regulation of sleep and wakefulness, physiological measurements associated with sleep, standard definitions of sleep architecture, and theoretical arguments of normal sleep function. This foundation of current knowledge regarding sleep characteristics will be valuable, as many explanatory approaches to insomnia incorporate evidence of established sleep abnormalities or even postulate malfunction in basic sleep-related physiological processes. Therefore, the contemporary basic measurements and theoretical models of normal sleep are important for comparison in several of the insomnia perspectives elaborated in the following chapters.

Sleep Happens

It is self-evident that whatever it is that we call sleep happens, and usually on a regular basis in a fairly predictable manner. We know that we sleep and that others around us sleep. The constellation of typical sleep-related behaviors is familiar and easily observed. Sleep can be described in behavioral terms that reflect the reversible state of characteristic body postures and decreased sensitivity to external stimuli. Normally, sleep feels refreshing, seemingly undoing sleepiness that may have been experienced before the commencement of the sleep episode. We normally have a sense of being about to fall asleep, and we are familiar with observing others falling into sleep. For instance, hearing the characteristic change in breathing pattern will inform a bed partner that the other has entered the transition into sleep, as would watching a fellow student nod off during a lecture.

Most people can take for granted that they naturally will sleep each night and that it will happen almost automatically. Like breathing, the regular cycle fortunately operates without required thought, but the pattern can be altered voluntarily or because of physiological demands. People may recognize the positive values of adequate sleep and the negative consequences of insufficient sleep, but nightly sleep usually occurs as a routine.

Rest and Activity

Fairly predictable variation in the level of certain types of activity occurs in all organisms, including bacteria and humans. Even many plants have intrinsic rhythms of approximately 24 hours. Invertebrates have clear 24-hour rest-activity cycles that typically are synchronized with the photoperiod (Tobler, 2000). It is within this context that the sleep-wake cycle, and its various functions, has evolved. Phylogenetic studies demonstrate that typical daily amounts of sleep vary among species but are fairly characteristic within species. The typical daily sleep quota for the elephant is about 4 hours, while that of the opossum is about 18 hours (Zepelin, 2000). Humans tend to sleep about 8 hours, with some sleeping much more and many others, especially in our society, sleeping considerably less.

How Much Is Enough?

The construct *sleep need* often is used, but rarely is it defined. The typical context is, "How much sleep do people need?" However, the need for *what* should be specified in formulating an answer. That is, an outcome influenced by sleep amount should be identified. Is the question about sleep need for optimal daytime alertness and performance, to remain healthy, to get by without dangerous consequences, or to survive? Individuals identifying themselves as suffering from insomnia may have concerns in all of these realms.

One approach to considering human sleep need is to examine how much people will sleep on a daily basis over a period of several weeks if there are a conducive environment and no schedule restrictions. After going to bed, subjects are allowed to sleep until they awaken spontaneously. Such a study can be done with healthy individuals who do not have disorders or take substances that might influence their ability to sleep or to remain awake. This should allow individuals to sleep as much as they need, if sleep need is defined as the amount that one will sleep on a regular basis if given the opportunity. Research of this sort was performed at the National Institutes of Health by Thomas Wehr and his team of investigators (Wehr et al., 1993). Their subjects, kept in darkness from dusk until dawn, stabilized at an average total daily sleep amount of about 8 hours and 15 minutes, after sleeping somewhat longer during the initial phase of the study, during which they presumably were making up for a mild sleep deprivation inherent in their previous schedules. The sleep during these long nights tended to be bimodal (i.e., divided into early and late sleep episodes). During the night they slept a few hours, were awake a few hours, and then slept a few more hours. These findings have implications relevant for some types of insomnia complaints and are discussed further in chapter 5.

Sleep need also can be addressed with research protocols that assess daytime sleepiness and an assortment of performance measures (e.g., reaction time, memory, and ability to perform tasks) in the context of schedules that allow only certain amounts of nighttime sleep. There is a general estimate that performance declines about 25 percent for every 24 hours without sleep. Higher cognitive processes, such as decision making, are much more sensitive to deterioration due to sustained sleep deprivation. Gregory Belenky and colleagues performed a study on men who lived in a research setting for a week and were assigned to groups that allowed them to be in bed each night for three, five, seven, or nine hours (Balkin et al., 2001). Of course, those with the shortest durations available for sleep were profoundly sleepy during the daytime and after one week fell asleep quite rapidly during test nap opportunities. Especially interesting was the finding that the subjects in the nine-hour sleep opportunity group objectively were less sleepy than those who were limited to seven hours in bed nightly during the previous week. This also suggests that the sleep need relative to optimal daytime alertness and performance is slightly greater than eight hours and therefore is longer than many individuals in our society allow themselves.

Usually sleep need is conceptualized as an amount of sleep required nightly on a regular basis. However, sleep need relative to the immediate danger of the intrusive sleepiness that might lead to inattention, and possibly to an accident, may depend on both acute and chronic sleep insufficiency. To a certain extent, sleep loss is cumulative over time, thereby leading to increasing potential impairment. For this reason, it is difficult to say how much sleep people require over the previous 24 hours to perform a task safely, since their sleepiness will be influenced by their sleep amounts during the previous days and weeks. Viewing recent sleep in terms of a running average over a period of several days is useful. The potential for impairment increases as this average sleep amount falls. In extreme circumstances of sleep insufficiency, any sleep is better than no sleep. Even a brief nap can offer temporary improvement in performance tests.

The idea of getting enough sleep to get well or remain healthy seems ageless and in the realm of common knowledge. In popular culture, lack of adequate sleep often is blamed for increasing one's susceptibility to illness. Unfortunately, estimating a precise sleep need with regard to general health or in relation to an absolute minimum necessary for survival is difficult. Sleep influences various physiological processes, including immune system functioning, and sleep loss may affect these adversely (Moldofsky, 1995). The exact amount of sleep loss over what time period required for identifiable pathology awaits further investigation. As for survival, no humans are known to have died directly from a lack of sleep (except from accidents due to sleep deprivation); however, death presumably related to fulminant infection has been demonstrated in animal studies, such as with rats typically not surviving longer than two to three weeks when prevented from sleeping (Everson, 1995).

Regulation of the Sleep-Wake Cycle

Two general processes are thought to influence the amount and timing of sleep under ordinary circumstances. These processes also affect the degree of sleepiness or alertness at any time of the day or night under any conditions. These two processes typically operate in concert, promoting the usual pattern of nighttime sleep and daytime alertness; however, they may be dissociated and, with some limitations, may be investigated independently. These two primary processes, termed the homeostatic and circadian, will be discussed separately and then together as they are integrated under circumstances of regulation of the sleep-wake cycle (Dijk and Edgar, 1999).

The Homeostatic Process

The homeostatic process reflects a pressure for sleep that results from the overall balance of sleep and waking. Accordingly, as people remain awake longer, greater pressure for sleep accumulates from this process. In fact, this homeostatic process might be considered as beginning from the moment of awakening and continuing until sleep occurs again. Normally, the homeostatic process should enhance the ability to fall asleep at one's habitual bedtime. However, purely from the homeostatic influence, the timing of sleep would not matter, as long as one was getting a sufficient amount of sleep. That is, one could sleep at random times and with various durations at any hour throughout the 24-hour day. Of course, that is not how most people exist, which is one reason it is evident that other factors also regulate the sleep-wake cycle. As noted above, the habitual sleep amount varies among species. For humans, the homeostatic drive for sleep seems to be about eight hours (one-third of the daily sleep-wake cycle). Sleep in some manner discharges the homeostatic pressure, thereby allowing subsequent alertness. Obviously, this balance occurs over a relatively short time period—just a few days. People cannot remain awake effectively for extended periods, nor can they sleep indefinitely. One cannot sleep continuously for one week and then remain awake the following two in order to satisfy the 1:2 ratio of sleep to waking.

Homeostatic sleep pressure generally represents the sleep need discussed above. This balanced drive for sleep can be seen as minimal during the daytime when people have been getting fully adequate nighttime sleep. It should be at a moderate level that enhances sleep onset as bedtime approaches. If a person is deprived of sleep, the homeostatic sleep pressure can cause a marked degree of sleepiness. Excessive sleepiness can result from acute sleep loss, chronic sleep insufficiency, or a combination of these. Such mixtures of sleep insufficiency are rather common in our society.

The Circadian Process

The circadian process is a manifestation of the internal circadian clock, which is an intrinsic biological rhythm. The term *circadian* refers to an approximate 24-hour rhythm and therein captures the important idea of flexibility of the periodicity. The rhythm may be slightly shorter or longer, depending on the individual species and the light-dark (photoperiod) timing, which can be manipulated under experimental conditions. In mammals it is organized through the activity of the rather small, paired suprachiasmatic nuclei (SCN) in the anterior hypothalamus (Zlomanczuk and Schwartz, 1999). Recent genetic studies have elaborated several genes (e.g., tau, tim, frq, clock, per) that direct transcription and create the circadian feedback loop within the neurons in the SCN (Wisor and Takahashi, 1999). While this approximately 24-hour rhythm in the SCN has its own internal momentum, there is external influence from the light-dark cycle by way of the retinohypothalamic tract. Most physiological parameters, including the core body temperature and a variety of hormonal processes, demonstrate fluctuation in relation to the normal day-night cycle, and many of these fluctuations persist in the absence of exposure to normal light-dark variation. The circadian system allows the synchronization of a multitude of physiological processes and bodily functions. An important feature of circadian oscillation is a certain degree of self-sustaining momentum. It takes time for the circadian system, and its associated influence on sleepiness, to adapt to new environmental stimuli. Rapid shifts can result in temporary desynchronization, as with jet lag.

The timing of the circadian system is apparent through measuring the fluctuation of such variables as the core body temperature and the level of serum melatonin. These can be conceptualized as hands of the clock. With appropriate manipulation of the exposure to light and darkness, the timing (phase) of the entire synchronized circadian system can be shifted. In a laboratory setting where all light and dark exposure can be controlled, the circadian system can be changed to any time, regardless of the actual external clock time. A phase-response curve demonstrates the influence of an independent variable on the phase of the circadian system, as represented by the core body temperature pattern or other manifestations of the intrinsic rhythm (Czeisler and Wright, 1999). The phase-response curve for the effect of light on the circadian rhythm in humans shows that exposure to light near the habitual time of sleep onset has a delaying influence on the rhythm, while light exposure near the habitual wake-up time has an advancing influence that shifts the cycle earlier. Toward the end of the normal sleep period, there is an inflection region of the curve, such that light exposure before that time delays the rhythm while light exposure after it advances the rhythm. The potency of the light in this phase-shifting influence is greater near either side of the inflection zone. This allows relatively dim dawn light to help maintain 24-hour entrainment in the human circadian system intrinsically running at a slightly longer periodicity. While these phase-shifting effects are demonstrated readily under experimental conditions, in real-life circumstances light and darkness at varying levels, durations, and timing may influence the circadian system in ways that may be beneficial or detrimental to one's desired sleeping and waking times.

The circadian process provides an underlying temporal organization for sleepiness and alertness and thereby for the timing of sleep and waking. That most people naturally tend to sleep at nighttime is neither random nor simply habit. From the homeostatic process alone, sleeping one out of every three hours could satisfy one's sleep requirement. However, human sleep gravitates toward nighttime. The regular routine reinforces the pattern, but it is driven primarily by the influence of the photoperiod (i.e., day-night cycle) on the SCN and its subsequent output. This alignment of the day-night and waking-sleep patterns occurs naturally; however, nighttime and sleep are not inextricably linked. Clearly, life circumstances create alternative schedules, although often these are not associated with ideal sleep. Sometimes the circadian system can become dissociated from the sleep-wake cycle. In the long-term temporal-isolation free-running studies mentioned below, some human subjects will shift to a longer sleep-wake period (e.g., sleeping for 11 hours and being awake for 22 hours) while the intrinsic circadian fluctuation of other physiological processes remains just over 24 hours. Because the circadian system has a limited range of entrainment, it is possible to dissociate the sleep-wake cycle from the circadian oscillation experimentally. This forced desynchrony can be achieved in laboratory settings where people follow a longer-than-usual sleep-wake schedule, as with a 28-hour "day." In such conditions the sleep episodes may vary somewhat, depending on where they fall with regard to the circadian cycle (Czeisler and Khalsa, 2000).

Research dating back many decades has shown that humans have circadian rhythms that are slightly longer than 24 hours. Long-term temporal isolation studies, performed initially in caves and later in research apartments without windows and clocks, have shown clearly this characteristic progressive delay in the sleep-wake pattern. Subjects live in these isolated settings for weeks to months. They remain completely unaware of the actual time and of whether it is daytime or nighttime outside. Interactions with the investigators and technicians are random to prevent clues about the outside time. The daily shift in the sleep-wake cycle when people are following their own body time represents the free-running pattern driven by the circadian system. Charles Czeisler and colleagues (1999) estimated the average human circadian period to be about 24 hours and 10 minutes. Figure 2.1 shows the typical pattern of sleep-wake cycle phase delay exhibited by humans in these long-term temporal isolation studies. Although the exact timing and duration of sleep may vary for each cycle, there remains a profound influence from the circadian system intrinsic period.

Under normal circumstances, when people are exposed to the day-night cycle, this circadian system generally is reset on a daily basis by the photoperiod; however, the slightly longer than 24-hour tendency is consistent with some common phenomena. For instance, most people find rapid westward travel over a few time zones easier to tolerate than going eastward. Staying up later and sleeping later, especially in accord with the photoperiod in the new time zone, is following the natural internal gradient. Rapid travel eastward, in a sense going upstream against the natural circadian tendency to delay, is more likely to result in symptoms of jet la

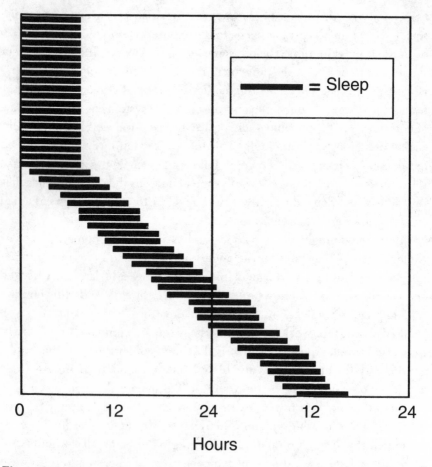

Figure 2.1 An example of a free-running pattern in a temporal isolation protocol. During the initial 20 cyles, the subject experiences typical external 24-hour influences (e.g., clock-determined daytime light and nighttime darkness), but for the subsequent cycles external input is removed. The sleep-wake pattern follows the intrinsic timing of the circadian system, which is slightly greater than 24 hours.

The direction of travel becomes less significant as more time zones are crossed and people become further out of synchronization with their new setting. The fundamental progressive phase-delay tendency in humans is also evident in the ease with which some people stay up later and subsequently sleep later during weekends and vacations. This can continue to the point where returning to a regular work schedule becomes challenging.

Integration

The homeostatic and circadian processes operate together in a complementary manner that normally optimizes the ability of people to sleep effectively for about 8 hours and remain awake and alert for about 16 hours. The ability to fall asleep at one's typical bedtime is enhanced by the homeostatic sleep pressure that has accumulated from being awake throughout the daytime. The intrinsic circadian sleepiness drive normally peaks toward the end of sleep period, typically about two hours before one's habitual spontaneous awakening time. Since homeostatic sleepiness is being discharged during the first few hours of sleep, later circadian sleepiness enhances continued sleep during the last few hours of the night. The opposite occurs during the daytime. Alertness during earlier daytime is facilitated by the low homeostatic sleepiness drive during this period. Conveniently, the circadian pattern of alertness peaks in the evening, just a few hours before one's habitual sleep-onset time. Low sleep propensity in the evening helps promote sustained alertness during the typical 16-hour wakeful period. On the other hand, attempts to sleep during this circadian phase may be frustrating and contribute to an insomnia complaint.

A common exception to the dichotomy of nighttime sleepiness and daytime alertness is midafternoon sleepiness that may result in a dip in alertness or even regular sleep episodes (e.g., siestas, "power naps"). This afternoon sleepiness is not inevitable, as adequate nightly sleep normally allows sustained daytime alertness. When people are even mildly sleep deprived, however, it is during the midafternoon that they are most likely to experience some difficulty remaining alert and awake. This vulnerability of increased afternoon sleepiness seems to be an intrinsic characteristic of the circadian system and is not primarily due to a midday meal (as the term *postprandial sleepiness* incorrectly would suggest). Although afternoon napping is facilitated by the circadian system, it may have significant homeostatic consequences. A nap may be beneficial in promoting alertness and improved performance during the next several hours; however, it may reduce the sleepiness necessary for rapid sleep onset at one's desired bedtime. A nap that is relatively early and short, perhaps about 20 minutes, is less likely to have detrimental effects. On the other hand, in the context of sleep deprivation, a longer nap will be beneficial. One additional potential problem with longer naps is the risk of feeling worse due to sleep inertia (see below, under "Electrophysiological Measurements").

Experimentally differentiating the respective sleep-promoting influences of the homeostatic and circadian processes is rather challenging, as both always are present. Evidence of the intrinsic circadian sleepiness drive can be derived from several different strategies. Studies of repeated opportunities for brief naps offer one reflection of the intrinsic sleepiness pattern. Another clever approach involves ultrashort day lengths that still allow one-third of the total time available for sleep. For instance, a "20-minute day" allows about 7 minutes for sleep (Lavie, 1989). The successive 13 minutes of waking and 7 minutes of sleep opportunity can be repeated over a 24-hour period or longer. The pattern of sleep amounts during the brief sleep opportunities will be influenced by the circadian sleep propensity. Roger Broughton (1994) demonstrated how the sleepiness patterns from very different research protocols tend to coincide. This composite pattern of the circadian sleep propensity is demonstrated in figure 2.2. The major nighttime and minor afternoon sleepiness peaks are evident, as is the low point in sleepiness in the early evening. The influence of this underlying circadian sleepiness pattern is consistent with typical real-life experiences, particularly the experience of an afternoon "slump" and then a "second wind" in the early evening.

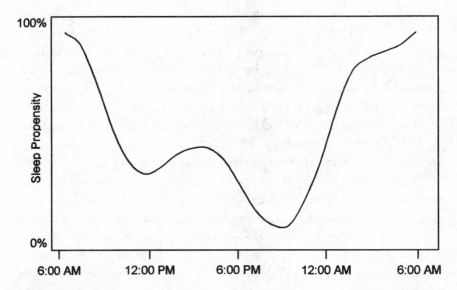

Figure 2.2 Estimate of the typical circadian-driven patterb of sleep propensity.
Source: Adapted from Broughton, 1994

This discussion of sleep-wake cycle regulation assumes maturity. The sleep propensity pattern of the human newborn lacks temporal organization. The average daily sleep of about 16 to 17 hours occurs relatively randomly. Very gradually over the first few months of life, sleep is more likely to occur during the nighttime. Some daytime sleep in the form of napping typically does continue during the first few years. Although the SCN is thought to be functional at birth, the entire circadian system, with its necessary input and output mechanisms, evolves only gradually during the first few months of life. This maturing circadian system is apparent from the increasing day-night differentiation of such parameters as the infant's core body temperature and melatonin secretion pattern. The sleep that occurred initially just from the homeostatic drive eventually is shaped by the significant influence of the circadian system, which, in turn, is influenced by the photoperiod.

Fundamentally, the homeostatic and circadian processes of sleep-wake regulation are presented as heuristic constructs. Although there are not yet precise explanations of how physiological mechanisms connect each process with the experience of sleepiness, these constructs are quite valuable in theoretical modeling, developing experimental protocols, explaining common experiences, and helping to identify the cause of many sleep-related clinical problems. The appreciation of this pronounced circadian sleep propensity pattern and the influence of homeostatic sleep pressure creates an important broad context for the complaints of sleepiness or sleeplessness at any particular time of the day or night.

Sleep and Brain Physiology

Although the sleep-wake cycle normally is synchronized with the physiological activity of various organ systems and most parts of the body probably benefit in some manner from regular sleep, it is clear that the primary sleep regulatory mechanisms and the key functions of sleep relate to the brain. Neuroanatomical and neurophysiological investigations during the past century increasingly have demonstrated that sleep is integrated throughout the brain in a complex manner. Normal sleep involves significant changes throughout the brainstem, midbrain regions, and cerebral cortex. The thalamus plays a major role in integrating signals across a wide range of frequencies, therein helping to regulate consciousness and levels of sleep. Most major neurotransmitters (e.g., serotonin, norepinephrine, histamine, acetylcholine, and gamma-aminobutyric acid [GABA]) and many neuropeptides, amino acids, and other brain substances vary considerably in relation to the sleep-wake cycle and different sleep stages. What once seemed relatively simplistic, such as the suggestion that increasing serotonin leads to sleepiness, soon became extraordinarily complex. Substances in the brain can have activities across spectrums of agonist, antagonist, and inverse agonist functioning and also can have more sustained modulatory roles. Further, the particular actions of brain substances can be highly localized and time dependent. Ultimately, it has become clear that sleep is an actively regulated and complicated function, thus leading to an appreciation of sleep as much more than simply the absence of wakefulness. While there are key localized sleep-related mechanisms, essentially sleep is a function integrated throughout the brain.

Electrophysiological Measurements

The activity of individual neurons generates electrical patterns due to the intracellular/extracellular charge differential and the action potential. Certain laboratory preparations allow the recording of single neurons or the activity of small regions of the brain. In rather limited circumstances, electrodes placed on the surface (electrocorticography) or within the human cerebral cortex (depth electrodes) allow precisely localized recordings. However, in human research and clinical studies, the EEG is a convenient method that offers a representation of the composite electrical activity of millions of neurons below a particular EEG lead. Soon after Hans Berger's development of the EEG in the late 1920s, it was used to examine brain activity during sleep. It was evident immediately that sleep was not a homogeneous state but rather was associated with a dramatic range of brain electrical activity. Different EEG patterns generally could be correlated with the depth of sleep, as reflected by observations and experimental arousal thresholds. Loomis, Harvey, and Hobart (1936) developed a system of sleep stages with criteria based on particular EEG wave patterns and the amount of slow-frequency electrical activity present. They suggested that greater slow-wave activity was associated with deeper sleep.

At different times and from different general brain regions, the EEG may record amplified neural electrical activity across a rather wide frequency spectrum and with a significant amplitude range. The frequency distribution typically is divided into bins, which are familiar because of their wide application. They are described in terms of the equivalent units of cycles per second (cps) or hertz (Hz). Although the precise boundaries of frequency bins may vary slightly with different systems, the typical standard demarcations of the EEG frequency spectrum, beginning with the slowest, are shown in table 2.1. The demarcations are somewhat arbitrary; however, they do represent useful clusters in describing brain activity in different stages of sleep and waking.

Standard EEG recordings typically incorporate filters that block out frequencies at the high and low ends of the frequency spectrum (Carskadon and Rechtschaffen, 2000). However, investigators may focus specifically on other ranges. For instance, there has been recent interest in very low frequency brain activity (below 1 cps) and in the spectrum from about 20 to 50 cps, which is termed the *gamma range*. In fact, the frequency bins can be abandoned entirely in certain research applications that use signal-processing formulas made possible on a large scale by digital technology. With these techniques it is possible to measure the degree of activity of any defined frequency range over a specified time period. For example, the mathematically calculated power of 1 to 2 cps activity per minute can be examined over an entire eight-hour sleep period.

The EEG signal amplitude may vary considerably with states of consciousness and among individuals. Children tend to generate signals of greater amplitude than do older adults. For an individual, the signal amplitude typically is greater at the lower end of the standard frequency spectrum. A primary reason is synchronization, wherein a pacemaker organizes simultaneous electrical patterns leading to the accumulation of the signal

Table 2.1   Typical EEG Frequency Bins

EEG Frequency	*Range in Hz*
Delta	0.5–3.9
Theta	4.0–7.9
Alpha	8.0–11.9
Sigma	12.0–13.9
Beta	14.0–19.9
Gamma	20.0–50.0

power. Recall that the amplified activity from a single EEG lead always represents a composite of the local neurons. During wakefulness, the neurons are doing many different things at the same time. During certain phases of sleep, numerous neurons are firing simultaneously. This is a normal phenomenon and is evident especially in what is termed *slow-wave sleep*. Pathological high-amplitude EEG patterns due to abnormal synchronous discharge commonly are observed in individuals with seizure disorders.

The current standardized system of sleep stages incorporates criteria from one or more EEG leads as well as activity recorded from electrooculogram (EOG) and electromyogram (EMG) leads (Carskadon and Rechtschaffen, 2000). Together, these leads represent the most basic polysomnogram (PSG) for scoring sleep stages, although other parameters (e.g., electrocardiogram, respiratory effort, oxygen saturation) typically also are monitored. The system was codified in 1968 (Rechtschaffen and Kales) and evolved from earlier reports of the EEG and sleep depth but incorporated new understandings of sleep physiology related to the phase of sleep that is termed *rapid eye movement* (REM) sleep. Polysomnographic records, typically representing an entire night, are evaluated in 30-second epochs, each of which is assigned a score of awake, REM sleep, or non-REM (NREM) sleep, the last of which must be specified further as stage 1, 2, 3, or 4. Movement artifact may be coded if signal interference makes the epoch impossible to designate. The duration of the PSG study, most typically a normal nighttime sleep period, can be described in terms of the amounts and percentages of waking and the individual sleep stages, and it can be graphed over time to create a visual representation of the progression of sleep stages throughout the recording time. The PSG is vital in the evaluation of several different sleep disorders, and it is an important tool for research regarding sleep.

The normal waking EEG typically will exhibit a mixed-frequency pattern with relatively low voltage, assuming the subjects have their eyes open or are attending to some mental activity. However, if they are relaxed with their eyes closed, then alpha activity often will predominate on the EEG, particularly in the occipital region. Typically, the sleep-onset transition is identified as relaxed wakefulness becomes light sleep, which is indicated by a disappearance of the alpha pattern and a general slowing of the background rhythm. There continues to be a low-voltage mixed-frequency pattern, but there also may be theta activity and sharp waves at the vertex. This light sleep represents NREM stage 1, and normally it lasts no more than a few minutes at the beginning of the sleep period. It may reappear for brief periods during a normal night. In certain circumstances, including some sleep disorders, however, there may be large amounts of NREM stage 1 sleep. Excessive light sleep measured on the PSG often corresponds with a subjective report of unrefreshing sleep and sometimes the sense of not having slept at all.

Aside from the changes in frequency and amplitude associated with levels of waking and sleep, other EEG complexes normally are encountered while monitoring sleep. Several of them have become integrated into criteria for sleep stages. These include the K-complex and spindles that are found during NREM stage 2 sleep. The K-complex is a distinctive, sharp, negative deflection followed by a positive component, together lasting up to 0.5 second. The spindles are EEG events lasting 0.5 to 1.5 seconds and having a frequency between 12 and 14 cps. As the name suggests, spindles have a characteristic shape with a gradual increase and then decrease in amplitude. Both K-complexes and spindles occur in the context of the typical NREM stage 2 background rhythm of mixed-frequency low-amplitude activity. Most people normally will spend at least one-half of their total nighttime sleep in NREM stage 2.

The EEG pattern evolves a dramatically different appearance when the rhythm slows and the amplitude increases due to thalamic pacemaker activity. Delta waves are identified when the frequency is below 4 cps and they meet the amplitude scoring criteria of at least 75 microvolts. This slow-wave activity occurs mostly during the first few hours of normal nighttime sleep, primarily before the first REM period and to a lesser extent between the first and second REM periods. The degree to which slow-wave activity is present varies considerably among individuals and is influenced strongly by age. Children tend to have high-amplitude and longer-duration slow-wave activity, which may account for 30 percent or more of their total sleep. With aging there is a gradual decline in the amplitude and duration of the EEG activity that would meet the criteria for NREM stages 3 and 4. It is not unusual for older individuals to have little or no slow-wave sleep. The designations of NREM stage 3 and stage 4 sleep are continuous and are based on the percentage of qualifying delta wave activity in each epoch. If more than 20 percent of the epoch consists of delta activity, then it is coded as NREM stage 3 unless the delta waves constitute over half of the epoch, in which case it is coded as NREM stage 4.

The slow-wave or delta EEG pattern is the key feature of NREM stages

3 and 4, and sometimes these stages together are termed *slow-wave sleep* (SWS) or delta sleep. In contrast to the highly activated brain states of wakefulness and REM sleep, the portions of NREM sleep where intense slow-wave activity predominates (i.e., relatively early during a normal night) reflect a different level of dynamic brain organization. In the terminology of chaos theory, this very regular SWS would be ascribed a rather low correlation dimension. Accordingly, the brain in SWS can be seen as lacking flexibility. Some people have difficulty quickly returning to agile alertness on awakening from sleep, especially after prolonged and intense slow-wave activity. This phenomenon is termed *sleep inertia*. Memory processing can be impaired, and there may be frank confusion. There is a common anecdote of people being awakened by a ringing telephone about one hour after sleep onset and then not recalling the conversation the following morning. Abundant slow-wave activity seems to play a role in the pathology of certain parasomnia sleep disorders, such as sleep terrors. The problem with feeling worse (e.g., mentally foggy, sluggish) after prolonged daytime napping is this sleep inertia, which becomes more likely as people sleep longer. Since SWS at nighttime is mostly early in the night, there still are several hours to recover from the effects. Compared with SWS, the only global brain activity with a lower level of organization, other than a completely flat line on the EEG, would be the highly regular pathological activity during a seizure. To a certain extent, there is a similarity between the postictal and sleep inertia states.

The NREM sleep stages are punctuated by REM sleep that occurs in distinct episodes totaling about 15 to 25 percent of normal nighttime sleep. The first REM episode typically emerges roughly 90 minutes after sleep onset, and REM sleep recurs about every 90 minutes. Usually, there are four to five episodes during a night. The REM episodes have a tendency to lengthen in duration as nighttime sleep progresses. Thus, the majority of REM sleep typically is during the latter part of the night. This aspect of the timing of REM sleep is influenced by the circadian system. The shift from NREM to REM and back is determined in the pons region of the brainstem, and it is regulated by the balance of cholinergic activity promoting REM and monoaminergic activity (norepinephrine and serotonin) promoting NREM (Siegel, 2000).

REM sleep is vastly different from NREM sleep. During REM sleep, the brain is in an activated state, somewhat similar to being awake but without the same input and output functions. Cerebral blood flow and certain metabolic activities are at the waking level. Although mentation may occur during any sleep stage, REM sleep is associated with active and sometimes intense dreaming. Other physiological changes include greater heart rate and blood pressure lability, markedly decreased thermoregulation, and the presence of penile tumescence. There is a remarkable skeletal muscle atonia during REM sleep. This results from a medullary process of active inhibition that prevents stimulation of the cerebral cortex motor area from being transmitted to the muscles. Accordingly, EMG leads register a decreased muscle tone associated with REM sleep. The other key feature of REM sleep is the presence of distinctive rapid eye movements, which are evident on the EOG tracing. The EEG activity during REM sleep is not particularly distinctive, in that it is a mixed-frequency, low-amplitude tracing, although sometimes there is a characteristic sawtooth pattern. This helps explain why it was two decades after the initial EEG sleep-scoring system before REM sleep was discovered. The data from the EOG and EMG are necessary for the identification and coding of REM sleep.

The hypnogram offers a convenient visual representation of a sleep period, typically a full-night PSG recording. Figure 2.3 shows a relatively normal night of sleep lasting about eight hours and incorporating the generally normal progression and amounts of sleep stages. There is considerable night-to-night and individual variation in the pattern, however, and the amounts of sleep stages are influenced strongly by age. Nevertheless, the hypnogram is quite useful in emphasizing the characteristic tendency for most SWS (NREM stages 3 and 4) to occur during the early hours of the night and for the recurrent REM episodes to lengthen in duration later in the night. A few brief awakenings identified by the PSG generally would be considered normal. Some abnormal patterns can be seen immediately on a hypnogram, such as a prolonged sleep-onset latency, early-morning awakening, frequent nighttime awakenings, and excessive NREM stage 1 sleep. In clinical sleep laboratory recordings, the resulting hypnogram also will show sleep-disordered breathing events and certain body movements, which can be correlated with the changes in the sleep stage.

The Body and Sleep

Although brain function is emphasized here, other organ systems demonstrate significant changes during sleep, in different sleep stages, and as

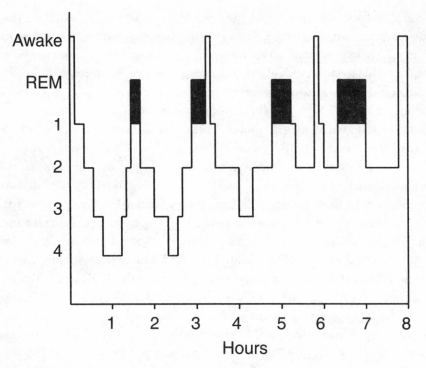

Figure 2.3 Hypnogram of sleep stages from a typical normal night of sleep in an adult human

part of a normal circadian oscillation synchronized with the sleep-wake cycle. There are clear alterations in thermoregulatory, cardiovascular, respiratory, and gastrointestinal physiological activity. A generalized parasympathetic predominance during NREM sleep is interrupted by autonomic swings during REM sleep. Dramatic endocrine changes are associated with sleep and circadian rhythms. This is evident particularly in the hypothalamic-pituitary axis. For instance, human growth hormone is secreted primarily during sleep, especially when SWS is most intense. Prolactin also is secreted mostly during sleep. Major circadian changes in cortisol and thyroid-stimulating hormone (TSH) normally occur during sleep. In each of these hormonal systems, changes with sleep (e.g., sleep deprivation) can influence the timing, pattern, and amount of the hormone released. Sleep also plays a role in the regulation of glucose levels. Even a moderate degree of sleep deprivation can lead to elevations on a glucose tolerance test (Spiegel, Leproult, and Van Cauter, 1999).

Accumulating evidence indicates that immune system function may be impaired with sleep deprivation. Accordingly, normal sleep may play an important role in maintaining host defenses on a regular basis. With infection, there often is an increase in the sleepiness drive. Immune mechanisms that promote recovery may be enhanced directly as a result of sleep (Moldofsky, 1995).

Normal sleep seems to be important for the cardiovascular system. During most of a normal night of sleep, there are significant reductions in heart rate and blood pressure. Both the lowered rate and afterload reduction seem to decrease the workload on the heart. This reduction of the blood pressure during the night seems to help maintain a normal daytime blood pressure in healthy individuals. It has been argued that severe sleep-disrupted breathing prevents the blood pressure drop and thereby contributes to the hypertension that is very common in this patient population.

The Functions of Sleep

Why is sleep so necessary? What functions does sleep serve? Why does sleep incorporate such diverse features as SWS and REM sleep? Currently, there are no firm answers to these questions, although accumulating research has led to exciting speculation about changes in brain chemistry during waking and sleep. Explanations of why sleep occurs have focused generally on such concepts as rest and restoration, energy conservation, and memory consolidation. There also are ecological arguments regarding temporal niches for species to maximize waking productivity (e.g., food acquisition) and sleep-time safety.

The idea that sleep has a role in energy conservation is particularly compelling, at least with regard to NREM sleep. From this point of view, sleep can be seen as helping to reduce energy consumption and perhaps resupplying brain energy constituents depleted during waking. Conceivably, the accumulation or depletion of key substances could contribute directly to the experience of homeostatic sleepiness. Other substances may be recycled. Glucose and oxygen use are decreased markedly during NREM sleep. While this alone may be advantageous, NREM sleep also may offer the opportunity for the repletion of energy stores. It has been suggested that brain glycogen is accumulated during NREM sleep. Adenosine also has been a focus of speculation regarding an energy-management theory of sleep. Clearly, adenosine has a vital energy role throughout the body by way of the ATP cycle. Adenosine antagonists, such as caffeine and theophylline, obviously inhibit sleep. Conversely, adenosine agonists seem to enhance sleep.

There has been widespread speculation about the functions of REM sleep, especially in relation to dreaming. There are multiple psychoanalytic and other psychodynamic explanations of why we dream. The unique physiological characteristics of REM sleep have stimulated other speculation. Since REM sleep has similarities with activity of the waking brain, it may represent an alerting mechanism. Perhaps REM sleep facilitates awakening in the morning. This would be consistent with the observation of little sleep inertia resulting from REM sleep awakenings and the fact that most REM sleep occurs toward the end of a normal night. REM sleep also has been seen as critical in brain development because fetuses, as well as newborns, spend great amounts of time in REM sleep.

The Realms of Disordered Sleep

Three very general but often overlapping symptom clusters lead people to seek help for their difficulties with sleeping. Most basically, these are too little sleep, too much sleepiness, and problematic behaviors during sleep. The complaint of not feeling able to sleep—insomnia—is the focus of this book. Insomnia is the most common sleep problem but not necessarily the most likely to prompt a visit with a health care professional. A diversity of processes contributing to the insomnia complaint is elaborated in the next four chapters. These include various psychological and physiological factors.

The expectation of normal sleep includes the assumption that one should be fully alert and free of excessive sleepiness during the waking hours. However, excessive sleepiness when one desires to be awake is a common difficulty and sometimes a major clinical problem. People with severe symptoms often do seek treatment, since sleepiness can interfere with daytime functioning. Excessive sleepiness most frequently is the result of sleep deprivation—acute or chronic. People sometimes are unaware that they do not allot sufficient time for adequate sleep, and they assume that some other problem must be accounting for their sleepiness and fatigue. However, certain sleep disorders certainly can cause daytime sleepiness that can range from mild to severe and that even can be life threatening in the context of driving or other situations of responsibility. With sleep-disordered breathing, there may be a normal amount of sleep; however, the quality of the sleep may be very poor. This may be indicated by a high percentage of NREM stage 1 sleep as well as reductions in SWS and REM sleep. In severe cases, the problem can be complicated by significant recurrent decreases in oxygen saturation levels. Some individuals exhibit frequent involuntary body movement during sleep, as with periodic limb movement disorder. These brief muscle contractions may be associated with arousals that decrease the quality of sleep and, in severe cases, can contribute to daytime sleepiness. Narcolepsy, a genetically influenced disorder with malfunction in the hypocretin (orexin) system, causes persistent daytime sleepiness as well as other symptoms reflecting abnormalities in REM sleep regulation. A variety of other pathological brain processes (e.g., traumatic, neoplastic, metabolic, and infectious) also may cause excessive daytime sleepiness. Finally, some medications and other substances can cause excessive sleepiness.

The third broad category of sleep disorders are the parasomnias, which are behaviors and abnormalities that emanate from sleep but are not primary problems of too much or too little sleep. However, patients with parasomnias may offer a chief complaint of insomnia when their sleep-related events cause annoying awakenings, or they may complain of excessive sleepiness when the parasomnia undermines their ability to achieve a sufficient amount of sleep. Some people with parasomnias are unaware of their sleep-related abnormalities and know of them only through other informants. The primary parasomnias include such phenomena as sleepwalking, sleep terrors, confusional arousals, nightmares, and REM behavior disorder. Being asleep also may increase the risk in vulnerable individuals for seizure activity, asthma episodes, arrhythmias, and panic attacks. Bruxism and enuresis may occur during sleep. The current understandings of sleep architecture described above are very helpful in differentiating the parasomnias, as several are associated with particular sleep stages. For instance, the dream-related anxiety of nightmares emerges from REM sleep. Slow-wave sleep is associated with confused behaviors occurring from sleep, especially with sleep terrors and confusional arousals.

The common denominator in this wide assortment of sleep-related complaints is that the experience deviates from the expectation of a normal sleep-wake cycle. People expect the ability to fall asleep quickly and remain asleep uninterrupted long enough (i.e., about eight hours) to feel fully alert during their waking hours. Wakefulness and sleep-disturbing behaviors should not intrude on sleep, and sleepiness should not intrude on wakefulness. Clearly, there are many reasons why this ideal fails to be achieved.

Summary

Insomnia exists only in comparison with what one considers to be normal sleep. With insomnia, sleep falls short of the expectation of how it should be experienced. People assess their sleep against a standard. However, normal sleep is relative. Various criteria and standards may be used to describe sleep as normal or abnormal. The approaches to examining sleep range from population epidemiology to individual physiology.

The sleep-wake cycle evolved in the context of the rest-activity cycle, which is evident to some degree in most living organisms. Humans naturally tend to sleep slightly more than eight hours daily, while other species may have shorter or longer sleep requirements. Homeostatic and circadian rhythm processes are important in the regulation of sleep under normal circumstances. The homeostatic process represents the total balance of sleep and wakefulness over time, while the circadian process reflects the entrained and synchronized physiological oscillation. Although typically entrained to the 24-hour day, the human circadian system intrinsically has a periodicity slightly longer than 24 hours. The homeostatic and circadian processes usually operate in concert; however, their influences can be dissociated in experimental or real-world circumstances.

A variety of physiological changes occur throughout the body in relationship to sleep and the circadian system. Brain activity, as represented by the EEG, varies greatly from waking to sleep and then during different stages of sleep. The EEG shows activity with considerable variation in frequency and amplitude, as well as some other distinctive wave complexes. A PSG recording incorporates the EEG, EOG, and EMG. Together these provide criteria for the standardized coding of sleep stages. The current sleep-staging system identifies REM sleep and four stages of NREM sleep. The generally normal progression of sleep stages during nighttime sleep can be represented graphically as a hypnogram.

There seem to be significant physiological benefits to various bodily systems from the regularity and sufficiency of sleep and circadian oscillations. Rest, restoration, and energy conservation probably are very important; however, there is increasing evidence of critical sleep-related regulation in hormonal, immunological, and cardiovascular systems. The lack of normal sleep may have many different consequences.

Although sleep generally is a vital aspect of the physiological functioning of humans and other higher organisms, there is no single, well-delineated function served by sleep. Clearly, it is necessary, but exactly why is not yet apparent. Several current theories focus on biochemical processes related to brain energy metabolism. Since NREM and REM sleep represent such different neurophysiological states with different levels of brain organization, presumably different needs are being met by the different sleep stages.

Most people do not complain about their sleep. However, the regulation of the sleep-wake cycle and of the stages of sleep is complex, and thus there is considerable potential for dysfunction leading to sleep disorders. Beyond intrinsic malfunction, a multitude of external factors can influence the experiences of sleep and waking. The most common sleep-related clinical presentations are complaints of not being able to sleep or of not being able to stay awake; however, people with parasomnias exhibit other abnormalities emanating from their sleep. All of these symptoms should be addressed in the context of the broad appreciation of processes normally regulating sleep and wakefulness.

3

Sleep as a Motivated Behavior

Insomnia results from a decreased drive of sleepiness.

The Motivated Behavior Perspective

The perspective of motivated behaviors delineated by McHugh and Slavney (1998) fosters an appreciation and understanding of symptoms that are influenced by physiologically driven and learning-reinforced behaviors. This view enhances our comprehension of a wide variety of normal and abnormal behaviors, and it can be an especially valuable tool in clinical situations. Many life problems may be formulated primarily in this realm of driven behaviors. The approach can highlight behaviors that vary with a range of drive intensity (insufficient, normal, excess) and with drive distortion or maladaptation that can result in abnormal expression. McHugh and Slavney point out that failure of treatment can result from inadequate recognition of these driven behaviors and learned habits. Intrinsic to the motivated behavior approach is the notion that treatment hinges on changing behaviors rather than curing diseases.

The concept of drive is the fundamental element of this perspective. Certain drives are essential components of life for both individuals and species. These include the physiological drives of hunger, thirst, sexual appetite, and sleepiness. Arousal and satiation of these drives are universal experiences that influence the behavior of all of us. It is rather challenging to imagine the human experience of our very earliest ancestors, but surely we share with them these identical basic drives and sensations.

Some behaviors associated with physiological drives can be viewed as preparatory or appetitive. These may involve activities, perhaps routines and habits, that lead to or support the desired ultimate consummatory behaviors. Food shopping and eating, courting and sexual intercourse, and lying down and sleeping all show this relationship. We may take these drives and related behaviors for granted, but with increasing deprivation the drive is enhanced and the behaviors are potentially more insistent. In extreme situations (e.g., starvation), deprivation can lead to an overwhelming focus on the satisfaction of the drive. Overall, the appetitive behaviors tend to be quite varied compared with the more stereotypic consummatory behaviors. While the behavioral expression of these drives typically is normal (i.e., healthy), clearly it is possible for problematic behaviors to result from abnormalities in these drives. Examples readily can be identified among the various eating, sexual, and sleep disorders.

Not so natural as the above examples, but still profoundly physiological, are the drives and subsequent behaviors that may be promoted by certain exogenous substances. Caffeine, nicotine, alcohol, opiates, and cocaine are clear examples. The social, economic, health, and legal ramifications of the presence of these substances in our society are staggering. In some cases the direct symptoms of physiological dependence strongly promote repeated consumption. This, in turn, necessitates a cascade of preparation—perhaps including robbery to obtain money for the next dose or simply stocking up on cigarettes. A routine cup of coffee in the morning may not be stimulated by a withdrawal headache or even by the daily worry that one might occur. Rather, for most people it is more a habit performed routinely without thought to the physiological drive. Cigarette smoking provides an excellent example of a drive that may be satisfied on a regular basis but intensifies dramatically in a withdrawal situation. The drive then is quickly satisfied with resumed smoking because of the highly efficient lungs-to-brain delivery of nicotine. The life consequences of these substance-related drives range from the trivial to the tragic. These driven preparatory and consummatory behaviors may, in fact, consume one's life.

McHugh and Slavney emphasize the drive, conditioning, and choice relationship inherent in the motivated behavior perspective. Drives influence behavior; however, considerable shaping or conditioning results from environmental, social, and cultural influences. These lead to the choices in behavioral responses. For instance, with the drive of hunger are a multitude of choices including when, where, what, and with whom to eat. Choices associated with sexual appetites range from no response to an assortment of potential behavioral expressions, which may or may not be culturally sanctioned. Sleeping behaviors also include a variety of potential responses to the underlying sleepiness drive.

Sleepiness: The Drive

Insomnia can be viewed as resulting from insufficient sleepiness or excessive arousal at the desired time of sleep. Accordingly, there may be fundamental underlying drive issues. Sleep presupposes the drive of sleepiness, whether naturally or unnaturally induced. Within limits, we are able to control whether we sleep; however, we have less control over whether we are sleepy. Under normal circumstances, this relationship of sleepiness and arousal promotes the typical pattern of daytime wakefulness and nighttime sleep according to the processes described in chapter 2. However, these can be altered by a wide variety of factors with the result of an inappropriate intensity or timing of sleepiness or arousal. Therefore, just as this perspective is valuable in viewing insomnia symptoms, it is equally applicable in the opposite circumstances of excessive sleepiness and irresistible sleep episodes.

Sleepiness is easily appreciated as a drive. The periodicity from the circadian oscillating system is obvious. It profoundly motivates our sleep behavior. Because of the homeostatic process, with sleep deprivation we become sleepier, ultimately to a point where sleep does become irresistible. Compared with other drives, sleepiness has a very high priority. Other satisfactions will be foregone or delayed in the presence of intense sleepiness. At times, sleep is our primary goal.

Behaviors promoted by the cycle of sleepiness include the ultimate consummation: sleep itself. However, many recurring routines or urgent appetitive behaviors readily are identifiable. For example, working backward from normal nightly sleep onset in one's home might be behaviors such as finding just the right position in bed, arranging pillows, saying prayers, a goodnight wish or kiss to a bed partner, turning off the lights, putting down a book or turning off the television, getting into bedclothes, brushing teeth and attending to other grooming activities, entering the bedroom at a regular evening hour—all directly or indirectly supporting the eventual realization of sleep. A more urgent appetitive behavior would be pulling into a rest stop for a nap after experiencing drowsiness during a long drive. Preparation for sleep obviously is important in light of our decreased ability to protect ourselves while in this mental state.

While there may be endless variations of these routines, they do, in fact, tend to be routine—followed in the same order most nights. The routines need not be promoted nightly by the direct experience of sleepiness but may represent learned behaviors with which we anticipate sleep and foster its occurrence. Some people remain active until they are unable to remain awake. They delay sleep onset until it becomes inevitable, ignoring the subtle cues of early sleepiness. Under normal circumstances, getting into bed and turning off the lights increases the probability of sleep onset, in contrast to interacting with a computer, walking a dog, or talking on the telephone at that same hour. A much more profound sleepiness must intrude on these activities to cause sleep compared with comfortably awaiting sleep while in bed. Generally, taking advantage of early sleep-onset opportunities will maximize sleep duration and minimize potential impairment resulting from excessive sleepiness.

How do we experience sleepiness? Sleeping is a paradoxical behavior in that we are not aware of it when we are doing it. This lack of awareness is a key defining characteristic of sleep. We are aware rather of wanting to sleep or of whether we have had sufficient sleep. We know that we have had a good or bad night of sleep after getting up in the morning. Sleepiness, in contrast with sleep, is felt directly, although subtly at times. We can explore both psychological and physiological aspects of sleepiness.

Sleepiness, of course, is associated with the desire to sleep. The lightest levels of sleepiness commonly are ignored. Therefore, the earliest time in the evening when one might fall asleep easily is delayed and perhaps not even noticed. Typical expressions of somewhat more intense sleepiness might include the following:

- I can't stay awake.
- I can't keep my eyes open.
- My eyes are itching and burning.
- I can't concentrate.
- I am fatigued and exhausted.
- I can hardly move.
- I wish I could lie down.

Sleepiness may be pleasurable or not depending on the circumstances. As one prepares to go to bed, one may anticipate and welcome a rapid sleep onset. In contrast, sleepiness will be unwelcome while driving or working late in a library on a project due the following day. Sleepiness ultimately will result in cognitive impairment, readily measurable in terms of memory, reaction time, and performance. It may be felt as a sense of mental sluggishness. Thoughts may be focused on finding a safe and comfortable place to achieve sleep quickly. Alternatively, circumstances might motivate one to pursue other strategies in the attempt to combat undesired sleepiness. Exercise, fresh air, and caffeine might be considered, although they will not necessarily achieve the desired effect of sustained alertness.

For both clinical and research purposes, questionnaires have been used to quantify aspects of the subjective experience of sleepiness. The Stanford Sleepiness Scale (Hoddes et al., 1973) inquires about the immediate level of sleepiness or alertness on a seven-item scale (exhibit 3.1). The Epworth Sleepiness Scale (Johns, 1991) takes a different approach in asking the responder to imagine the likelihood of falling asleep in eight defined circumstances (exhibit 3.2). Therefore, the Epworth scale should reflect a longer-term assessment of sleepiness. With both of these instruments, the measure of sleepiness can be reduced to a single number and can be used for comparative purposes.

Physically, sleepiness may include a feeling of weakness and fatigue and sometimes a sense of not wanting to move. Many people also describe sensations around their eyes in association with sleepiness. There may be a feeling of not being able to keep the eyes open; however, often there is a greater discomfort, described as a burning or itching. A localized increase in skin temperature around the eyes in association with sleepiness has been described (Niedermeyer, Jankel, and Uematsu, 1986). Curiously, allergy symptoms of eye discomfort may be perceived as sleepiness. Per-

---

Exhibit 3.1 The Stanford Sleepiness Scale

Circle the *one* number that best describes your level of alertness or sleepiness right now.

1. Feeling active, vital, alert, wide awake
2. Functioning at a high level but not at peak, able to concentrate
3. Relaxed, awake but not fully alert, responsive
4. A little foggy, let down
5. Foggy, beginning to lose track, difficulty in staying awake
6. Sleepy, prefer to lie down, woozy
7. Almost in reverie, cannot stay awake, sleep onset appears imminent

The SSS score is the single item number.

Source: Adapted from Hoddes et al., 1973

Exhibit 3.2 The Epworth Sleepiness Scale

How likely are you to doze off or fall asleep, in contrast to feeling just tired, in the following situations? This refers to your usual way of life in recent times. Even if you have not done some of these things recently, try to work out how they would have affected you. Use the following scale to choose the most appropriate number for each situation:

0 = would *never* doze
1 = *slight* chance of dozing
2 = *moderate* chance of dozing
3 = *high* chance of dozing

_____ Sitting and reading

_____ Watching TV

_____ Sitting, inactive in a public place (e.g., a theater or a meeting)

_____ As a passenger in a car for an hour without a break

_____ Lying down to rest in the afternoon when circumstances permit

_____ Sitting and talking to someone

_____ Sitting quietly after a lunch without alcohol

_____ In a car, while stopped for a few minutes in traffic

The ESS score is the sum of the individual items and ranges from 0 to 24.

Source: Adapted from Johns, 1991

haps the eyes are to sleepiness what the stomach is to hunger and the genitals are to sexual desire. All these drives are global, with brain direction and major cognitive components—but each has some degree of localized physical sensation associated with the desire and relieved with satiation.

While we typically consider sleepiness as a subjective experience, there must be physiological correlates. Sleepiness should reflect the propensity for sleep, or the likelihood of falling asleep. The degree of sleep propensity can be considered at any point in time, and sequential measurements should demonstrate the influence of the homeostatic and circadian processes, as well as the temporary sleep inertia mentioned in chapter 2. Sleep propensity can be measured objectively in how rapidly one falls asleep in a conducive setting (e.g., a comfortable bed in a relatively dark and quiet room). This is the basis of the Multiple Sleep Latency Test (MSLT), which is used widely in clinical sleep medicine (Thorpy 1992).

The MSLT typically is a daytime test performed after a nighttime sleep laboratory evaluation. The MSLT involves allowing an individual four to five brief nap opportunities at two-hour intervals during the day beginning about 9:00 A.M. Factors promoting sleepiness will result in a shorter average sleep-onset latency during the daytime naps. Usually, an average MSLT sleep latency of five minutes or less is considered to be a severe degree of sleepiness and may indicate a pathological process. Clinically, the test is performed as part of the evaluation of excessive sleepiness that may result from certain sleep disorders, such as narcolepsy or sleep-disordered breathing. Of course, the increased homeostatic sleep pressure resulting from sleep deprivation will shorten the sleep latency, so the recent sleep history is vital in interpreting the MSLT results. A variation of the MSLT, the maintenance of wakefulness test (MWT) (Mitler, Gujavarty, and Browman, 1982), calls for the subject to try to remain awake during nap opportunities, therein offering a reflection of potential impairment associated with daytime functioning. Although these standardized measures of sleep propensity have valuable clinical roles, the tests and similar strategies that measure the latency of sleep onset at various times are important research tools to measure circadian and homeostatic influences and to identify other physiological correlates of sleepiness.

The physiological measure defining sleep-onset latency in clinical nighttime and daytime sleep studies, as well as in most sleep research investigations, is the character of the amplified electrical activity from one or more electroencephalogram (EEG) channels. Frequency and amplitude on the EEG are easily observable and measurable, and recent digital technology allows more complex analyses of the electrical signal. As noted in chapter 2, wakeful relaxation and arousal are associated with varying degrees of alpha and beta activity on the EEG; however, even faster frequency ranges have been posited to have essential roles in attention and concentration (see table 2.1). The standard electrophysiological criteria for sleep onset include a slowing of the basic EEG rhythm into the theta range and perhaps down to the delta frequencies. These EEG changes roughly correlate with our familiar behavioral observations of sleep onset: relaxed posture, eyes closed, regular breathing pattern, and decreased responsiveness. The occurrence of these sleep-related EEG characteristics during wakeful activities certainly reflects sleepiness. Nodding off while sitting on the sofa in the evening may be benign, in contrast to the intrusion of these EEG theta "micro-sleeps" and lapses in attention while driving at 65 mph.

Are there any tightly correlated physiological measures of subjective sleepiness other than the conventional EEG? Generally, sleepiness follows a circadian pattern, which inherently incorporates a myriad of varying parameters. Accordingly, the core body temperature and pattern of melatonin secretion usually are correlated with the trends of sleep and sleepiness. The greatest circadian sleepiness corresponds with the low point in the rhythm of core body temperature. However, profound sleepiness and sleep onset can occur independently of these rhythms, so they do not represent the final links in the sleepiness experience.

Other strategies that have been used to measure sleepiness objectively are pupillometry (Yoss, Moyer, and Hollenhorst, 1970) and measurements of eye blink rate (Santamaria and Chiappa, 1987). With increasing sleepiness, there are increased pupil oscillations during adaptation to darkness. Sustained pupil dilation indicates autonomic activity associated with arousal. The eye blink frequency slows with sleepiness. Devices have been developed to measure the eye blink rate as an indicator of sleepiness. Rather sophisticated devices have been developed as sleepiness alarms to alert long-distance drivers and other people in situations requiring sustained alertness when they may be at risk for dangerous inattentiveness or actually falling asleep. These have incorporated such measures as eyelid droops over the pupil and patterns of heartbeat, respiration, and activity. Instruments of this type are especially valuable, as they can passively monitor the subjects in real-life circumstances. Even more sensitive assessments of sleepiness are possible with laboratory-based strategies involving subjects responding to stimuli under experimental conditions, including various schedules of sleep deprivation. David Dinges described a behavioral assay for sleepiness using a computerized vigilance test that measures how quickly subjects respond by pushing a button after repeated, randomly timed stimuli (Dinges and Powell 1985). The analyses can show abnormally delayed or missed responses, as well as those made incorrectly without a stimulus.

Research studies that induce sleepiness through scheduled sleep deprivation clearly demonstrate the cognitive impairment that accompanies the progressive lack of sleep. This has been shown most dramatically with continuous sleep deprivation over several days but is also readily demonstrated with restricted amounts of nightly sleep during a period of successive days. Extreme sleepiness is achieved after 2 to 3 days of complete sleep deprivation and is quite pronounced in the rare studies where humans have remained awake up to 10 days (Gulevich, Dement, and Johnson, 1966).

The mental effects may include irritability, attention and concentration deficits, decreased reaction time, and visual misperceptions and illusions. Extraordinarily severe sleep deprivation may result in visual hallucinations, grandiose and paranoid delusions, and confusion. There may be an increased startle response, nausea, and ataxia. Eye movement control may be impaired, resulting in blurred and double vision. Research study subjects may search desperately for unauthorized opportunities for sleeping. These sleep deprivation studies document the potentially dangerous performance impairment that ultimately will accompany increasing sleepiness in real-world situations where sleep deprivation is sometimes a routine part of everyday life, such as in the military and health care workers. The public health implications are great.

Aspects of sleepiness also are revealed in research studies focused on the sleep-onset period, that is, the transition from waking to sleep. A major conclusion of investigations in this area is that there is no single moment of sleep onset: falling asleep is not an instantaneous event (Rechtschaffen, 1994). Different measured parameters may meet the criteria associated with sleep onset at different moments. Measurable phenomena include the standard electroencephalographic recordings, tracings from implanted electrodes, ocular movements, responsiveness to various external stimuli, behavioral observations, cognitive test performance, and the perception of being awake or asleep. Sleep onset may best be viewed as a coordinated process, as opposed to a single instant in time.

In recent years it has become evident that, in addition to the obvious cognitive deficits, there are physiological consequences of sleep deprivation. While these effects parallel increasing sleepiness, it is not clear that there is a direct connection—they may result from independent sleep-related mechanisms. The most convincing evidence thus far has been in the areas of immune and endocrine function, especially as demonstrated in the research of Harvey Moldofsky (1994) and Eve van Cauter (2000). The close relationship of growth hormone secretion and sleep has been known for many years: sleep deprivation decreases the release and alters the secretion pattern. More recently, impaired glucose utilization has been demonstrated with sleep deprivation. The immune response to antigens also is compromised with sleep deprivation. The implications of these processes are yet to be fully explicated.

A compelling research question for more than a century has been whether there is a circulating humeral substance that induces sleepiness. The underlying issue relates to the substrate of the homeostatic sleepiness process, that is, what actually happens in the body during wakefulness that ultimately causes sleepiness. It has been hypothesized that a substance builds up systemically or in the brain during waking and produces sleepiness, thereby increasing sleep propensity. Presumably, this substance would be recycled through sleep. For many years experiments have been performed where animals have been deprived of sleep and then blood or cerebrospinal fluid (CSF) extracts have been isolated and injected into non-sleep-deprived animals. In recent years these types of studies have suggested that cytokine substances may have a critical role in driving sleepiness. James Krueger has shown that sleep and immune systems share regulatory molecules (Krueger and Fang, 2000). It also has been argued that particular brain metabolic pathways involving adenosine and/or glycogen are fundamental to the sleepiness drive. More recently, the neuropeptide hypocretin has been implicated in having a primary role in the regulation of sleep and arousal (Mignot 2000).

In summary, sleepiness promotes a constellation of behaviors that ideally enhance the opportunity for safe and adequate sleep. We regularly experience the arousal and satiation of the sleepiness drive. It motivates how we spend a substantial part of our lives. Humans experience a homeostatic sleep pressure for about 8 hours of sleep out of a 24-hour day, and the circadian system helps organize the timing of sleepiness and the likelihood of sleep, whether it is voluntary or involuntary. When and where we sleep further conditions our sleep-wake cycle because of influences on the homeostatic and circadian systems. These processes in turn contribute to our level of sleepiness or alertness in the near future. Individual choices and behavior can promote a regular pattern of daytime alertness and nighttime sleepiness or they can undermine the system, causing the inability to sleep adequately at a desired time.

The Balance Analogy

In addition to the homeostatic and circadian processes, a myriad of other factors can influence whether one is awake or asleep at any particular time. Multiple factors may promote arousal or sleepiness acutely or chronically.

Longer-term processes regulate our usual daytime waking and nighttime sleep; however, under certain circumstances, arousal suddenly can interrupt sleep, as can sleep intrude on the waking state. A simplistic balance analogy with factors promoting sleepiness on one side and arousal on the other is shown in figure 3.1. This balance model can help organize influences on the normal sleep-wake cycle and elaborate those factors inappropriately causing arousal or sleepiness at undesired times.

The normal cycle of sleep propensity, influenced primarily by the homeostatic and circadian processes, is reviewed in chapter 2. These two influences can be considered throughout the normal 24-hour cycle by the degree to which sleepiness or arousal is promoted. Sleepiness is expected at nighttime, first from the homeostatic pressure of being awake during the daytime and later due to the circadian sleepiness peak toward the end of the normal sleep period. Ideally, then, during the nighttime sleep hours, factors contributing to sleepiness should be pronounced and outweigh the arousal side of the balance. The opposite should be true during the daytime and early evening, with arousal outweighing sleepiness. In the daylight morning hours, arousal prevails as the homeostatic sleep pressure has been discharged with the previous nighttime sleep. The circadian system promotes maximum arousal in the early evening. Together these processes allow for the 16 hours of daytime and evening wakefulness. The balance may easily shift back temporarily in the midafternoon because of the underlying pattern of sleep propensity. Therefore, sleep probability increases, especially when there is higher homeostatic sleep pressure. Accordingly, early to midafternoon sleepiness is more likely to be a problem if one already is sleep deprived.

This motivated behavior balance model predicts that bedtime sleeplessness, and, therefore, the complaint of insomnia, may result from an insufficient sleepiness drive, excessive arousal, or a combination of these

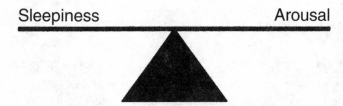

Figure 3.1　Sleepiness-arousal balance

two processes. The opposite also may be predicted: daytime sleepiness (and perhaps sleep itself) may be due to factors promoting decreased arousal or excessive sleepiness.

The complaint of insomnia may be entirely predictable based on this balance model. A long afternoon nap uses up homeostatic sleep pressure, so it is not available to aid sleep onset at a normal bedtime. Attempting to go to sleep a few hours before one's normal sleep-onset time may have the person in the zone of minimum circadian sleepiness and therefore at greatly decreased likelihood of falling asleep. A dessert espresso drink after dinner enhances arousal and decreases the probability of sleep within the next few hours.

The circadian contribution to the sleepiness side of the balance depends on the time of day, with the major peak near the end of the sleep period and the minor peak in the afternoon. Most people share a general entrainment with the photoperiod; however, there may be some schedule-related exceptions. Jet lag, shift work schedules, and circadian rhythm disorders are common examples of circadian-influenced sleep-wake problems, which will be explored further in this and subsequent chapters. The homeostatic contribution to sleepiness is derived from the duration of prior wakefulness and the overall degree of sleep deprivation, based on recent sleep history. An assortment of medical, psychiatric, and underlying sleep disorders also may contribute to the level of sleepiness. Included among the various factors that may influence the sleepiness-arousal balance at any particular time of day are those outlined in table 3.1.

Sleeping and waking always are influenced to some degree by the homeostatic and circadian processes. Other intrinsic and extrinsic elements also may shift the balance further one way or the other. Consider the situation of a large percentage of adults in Western industrial societies who are mildly chronically sleep deprived (getting a daily average of six and one-half to seven hours of sleep) and dependent on daily consumption of caffeine-containing beverages for daytime alertness. Also surprisingly common are circumstances where scheduled sleep and waking times are not coincidental with an individual's underlying circadian patterns of sleepiness and arousal. Jet lag includes obvious circadian influences, although homeostatic sleep loss often accompanies travel and contributes even further to the experience of jet lag. Below are various case examples of individuals complaining of insomnia that may be understood within the context of the motivated behaviors perspective.

Table 3.1 Arousing and Sedating Factors

Arousing	Sedating
Medication effects—stimulating	Medication effects—sedating
Alcohol—withdrawal effects	Alcohol—acute effects
Cocaine and some other illicit drugs	Heroin and some other illicit drugs
Selected medical disorders (e.g., hyperthyroidism, pheochromocytoma)	Selected medical disorders (e.g., hypothyroidism)
Selected psychiatric disorders	Selected psychiatric disorders
Selected sleep disorders	Selected sleep disorders
Caffeine	
Nicotine	
Pain, discomfort	
Excessive light or noise, temperature extreme	
Exercise—acute effects	
Emotional state: anxiety, fear, depression, excitement	

Insomnia in the Context of Motivated Behaviors

Napping

Napping, of course, is sleeping and therefore it discharges homeostatic sleep pressure. The consequences may be good, bad, or neutral. Napping is not necessarily a problem or a habit to be avoided. Napping may be an enjoyable part of one's daily routine. It may be life saving in circumstances of sleep deprivation. A brief "power nap" may be energizing and may enhance one's productivity. The tendency to nap in the early to midafternoon is not random coincidence. As discussed in chapter 2, the circadian and homeostatic systems create the increased proclivity for sleepiness during these hours. Even mild sleep insufficiency is likely to promote the familiar afternoon dip in alertness. Napping is the norm in siesta cultures. For some individuals, combined daytime and nighttime sleeping may be the ideal solution to achieving adequate total daily sleep.

On the other hand, napping may steal away the sleep pressure needed at bedtime to promote a reasonably rapid sleep onset. Through trial and error, many people realize the potential cost of napping in terms of worsened nighttime sleep. However, giving in to the temptation to nap (i.e., to behave in a manner to allow sleep in response to the motivation of sleepiness) ultimately can result in a vicious cycle: decreased nighttime sleep leading to increased daytime sleepiness and napping, then leading again to the nighttime inability to sleep adequately. This pattern can continue indefinitely with daytime and nighttime impairment and an overall decreased quality of life. The following case is an example of this nap trap.

John was a 45-year-old man who had had no sleep-wake complaints for most of his life. Typically, he slept soundly from about 10:00 P.M. until 6:00 A.M. For about 15 years he had a stable manufacturing position working a shift from 7:00 A.M. until 3:00 P.M. He lived close to the plant, so he was able to get to work and home again quickly. One year before his evaluation at the Sleep Disorders Center, reorganization at work required him to spend three months working the second shift (3:00 P.M. until 11:00 P.M.). He was unable to get to bed until around 1:00 A.M. He would fall asleep quickly but awaken spontaneously at about 6:00 A.M. Within the first week he found that he persistently felt tired. He began drinking coffee in the afternoon at work to help him remain alert. During the second week he began napping in the early afternoon before going to work and on his days off as well. He was delighted with the news that he could return to his preferred 7:00 A.M. to 3:00 P.M. shift. However, the transition back was not as smooth as he had hoped. He remained fatigued much of the time. He found some relief by napping for 60 to 90 minutes right after getting home from work in the afternoon. Instead of being able to fall asleep by 10:00 P.M., as he had previously, now he was frustrated by his inability to fall sleep until at least midnight. Either he would get in bed around 11:00 P.M. and then toss and turn for over an hour, or he simply would stay up watching television until after midnight and eventually go to bed and fall asleep by 1:00 A.M. He continued to drink coffee at work to try to combat his fatigue and poor concentration. He remained aggravated about his inability to fall asleep early enough at nighttime and his difficulty remaining fully alert and energetic during the daytime. He was also frustrated that his daily napping took away time that previously he had enjoyed with his family.

Three major factors are evident in this shift work case: circadian phase, homeostatic sleep pressure, and stimulation from caffeine. By history, John was predisposed to an early awakening. This was ideal for his initial shift schedule. When it became necessary for him to go to bed later, his circadian system did not allow him to compensate by sleeping later into the daytime. Significant sleep deprivation evolved, causing his poor concentration and ultimately the napping routine. While the napping was helpful for his functioning during the second shift schedule, the pattern had become entrenched by the time he switched back to the first shift. He had never broken free of the cycle of nighttime insomnia and daytime sleepiness. During his months working the second shift, he had used caffeine to help him remain awake at work, but he continued to do the same at home, thereby contributing to his late sleep onset. After behavioral changes, which included reorganization of his time appropriated for sleep and reduction in his caffeine consumption, he was able to return to a satisfying experience of daytime alertness and nighttime sleep.

This case demonstrates the problems encountered by an individual after an extended change in shift work schedule and the subsequent return to his original schedule. Even more disruptive, of course, are the effects of rotating shift work schedules, where people never have the opportunity to stabilize their internal and external clocks. There may be perpetual desynchronization and sleep insufficiency, resulting in pervasive impairment in quality of life.

An additional potential problem of napping is the sleep inertia that can evolve with prolonged sleep during a nap. Some people find that a short nap is energizing and refreshing and that a longer nap makes them feel mentally sluggish and generally worse physically. As suggested in chapter 2, sleep inertia may result from the slow-wave EEG activity that would be more likely to occur with longer sleep duration.

Shift Schedules

The circadian and homeostatic processes work well together under normal circumstances. Abnormal situations, such as shift work and other schedules that alter the hours available for sleep and wakefulness, undermine effective sleep and waking for predictable reasons. Trying to remain alert while working throughout the night, when the circadian system is promoting maximum sleepiness, is challenging, as is trying to achieve adequate sleep during the daytime, while the circadian system is promoting alertness. Shift workers commonly complain of the inability to get enough sleep. The problem is not necessarily having enough time to sleep but rather being in the right circadian zone for effective sleep. Shift workers remain exposed to the same photoperiod influences that reinforce nighttime sleep. Leaving work in the morning, they are exposed to the same morning light that entrains people who have just slept all night. Even workers doing permanent all-night shifts rarely adapt fully to the schedule. Understandably, they do not stick with the unnatural schedule on days off, and curtail daytime sleep opportunities for various activities (e.g., laundry, banking, shopping, car repairs, and socializing). Our increasingly on-line society is probably beneficial for some of these necessities, at least up to the point where it may offer new distractions and tempt one from sleep.

William was a 53-year-old man who presented to the Sleep Disorders Center with the complaint that he was unable to get enough sleep during the daytime. He was puzzled that he could not sleep all day, as he lived alone and generally there were no outside disturbances. Previously, he had slept well for about eight hours at nighttime. He had worked night shifts occasionally and recovered well within a night or two. He was employed as a care provider at a group home for emotionally disturbed youths. He explained that he had been working for 53 nights straight and that he had just gotten off work before coming in for his evaluation. Staff shortages had prevented any time off during this extended period. He was required to remain awake during the night. His responsibilities included working the hours from 8:00 P.M. through 8:00 A.M. He then would return to his home and get in bed by 9:00 A.M. He had little difficulty falling asleep but rarely remained asleep past early afternoon. At that point he would eat and attend to various chores before finally returning to the group home for another night. He estimated that he was getting four to five hours of sleep per day. During his waking hours he felt very fatigued, and he believed that he was not able to manage his supervisory role well under the current circumstances.

This man previously had been able to recover from the occasional stress of working the nightshift, as he generally was achieving sufficient sleep on the other nights. During this extended nightshift schedule, however, he never was able to catch up because of his inability to achieve sufficient daytime sleep. For him, it was not simply a matter of inadequate opportunity or desire but rather insufficient sleepiness. The consequences for him were rather debilitating. He was again able to function well soon after returning to his previous work schedule. Clearly, the mismatch of the imposed schedule and sleep propensity is the root problem and suggests the ideal solution. However, some people may benefit from the use of short-acting hypnotics to maximize the ability to sleep during hours of lower circadian sleep propensity.

Jet Lag

The term *jet lag* describes a constellation of symptoms resulting from various factors, including rapid transmeridian travel. Since the circadian system takes several days to readjust to a new photoperiod, the sleepiness and arousal promoted by the circadian clock occur at inconvenient times. The familiar symptoms are insomnia during the new desired sleep hours and sleepiness and fatigue when one desires to be awake and active. Mild sleep deprivation commonly is a contributing factor. Frequently, the problem is exacerbated by pretravel sleep loss as people stay up late packing and then get up extra early for airline flights. There may be other homeostatic issues. Some people invariably sleep on flights, perhaps in part because of the drone and relative immobility. If that occurs during the daytime, it may further reduce subsequent nighttime sleepiness. In contrast, some people can never sleep on flights, even when it is desired during nighttime "red eye" schedules. Other aspects of travel fatigue may result from the flight-related noise, vibration, low humidity, and immobility.

> Marie was a 34-year-old woman who worked for an international public relations company. Most nights she slept well; however, she knew that any sort of stress in her life could affect her sleep for at least a few nights. For two years her job had required her to travel to Europe once or twice a month for three to four days each trip. She enjoyed this travel initially but had come to dread each trip as she anticipated feeling miserable while there and for several days after returning home. Although her business travel often took her to different cities, she now avoided socializing and sightseeing. She felt that she never could get adequate sleep during her travel, and she felt that her work-related productivity and creativity were blunted. By the time she had fully recovered and felt normally rested, energetic, and mentally sharp, it was almost time for another trip. Her fantasy vacation now was staying home.

It was unfortunate that Marie could not simply stay in Europe for a few weeks or months at a time. Her circadian system could then adapt to the new time zones, and she would have the opportunity to enjoy herself, not feel so stressed about her travel, and probably be more effective with her work projects. She did experience some benefit with the occasional use of short-acting hypnotic medication for a few days. Ultimately, she was able to reduce the frequency of the international travel.

Circadian Zone Insomnia

The level of sleepiness and the ability to fall asleep vary considerably throughout the 24-hour cycle, primarily because of homeostatic and circadian influences. One typical element of the cycle is the low point in sleep propensity, sometimes described as a zone of wake maintenance or forbidden sleep (Lavie, 1989), which occurs naturally for most people in the early evening. Accordingly, attempts to fall asleep during this phase of low intrinsic sleepiness can be met with failure and frustration, as well as confusion about why sleep is not occurring. A predictable result may be the complaint of insomnia, which can occur acutely. For example, someone habitually falling asleep at 11:00 P.M. may decide to try going to sleep at 8:00 P.M. in anticipation of an early-morning flight and worry about rush-hour traffic. Unless this person already is significantly sleep deprived and therefore has considerable homeostatic sleep pressure, he or she probably will have great difficulty falling asleep at this early hour. Because of the relatively high intrinsic level of arousal still present, even the use of a hypnotic medication that early in the evening may not easily foster sleep onset.

Delores was a 45-year-old woman who lived alone and worked as a supermarket cashier. She had a stable work schedule from 8:00 A.M. until 4:30 P.M. She had had difficulty getting to sleep and staying asleep all of her adult life. She felt that she got her deepest sleep around the time her alarm clock awakened her at 6:45 A.M. On days she was not working, she would sleep until about 8:00 A.M. She never felt fully refreshed during the daytime, and working through the midafternoon always was a struggle for her. With hopes of giving herself the opportunity to get as much sleep as possible, she would get in bed by 8:30 P.M. She turned off the telephone ringer, shut off the lights, and got in bed. She never felt sleepy at this time. She attempted to relax and think positive thoughts, although she often ended up worrying about how she would feel and function the following day. She estimated that it usually took at least two hours before she initially fell asleep. She then would have a few awakenings before 2:00 A.M. After that, she usually stayed asleep until the alarm clock rang or her spontaneous awakening in the morning. She worried that if she went to bed later, it still would take her a few hours to fall asleep and she would feel much worse the next day.

This woman expected to be able to sleep, and she believed that she needed to be sleeping at a time when she was not sleepy. She was able to sleep much better when she went to bed at 10:00 P.M. She was much less anxious about going to bed when she found that she was able to fall asleep relatively quickly. Education regarding sleep-wake patterns and behavior changes were key elements in her treatment.

Blind Free-running

Generally, our circadian systems are entrained by the photoperiod. For humans, the endogenous clock has a period slightly longer than 24 hours, and the system is reset more or less on a daily basis. Most people tend to be "tuned" to dawn; that is, they awaken naturally for the day around dawn and typically become sleepy about eight hours before that time. Researchers have demonstrated that some blind individuals with no light perception will "free run" with their own intrinsic circadian period, since they do not have the opportunity for light entrainment (Sack et al., 2000). Their circadian systems, including the underlying rhythm of sleepiness and alertness, persist regardless of the actual clock time. The result may be a highly predictable pattern of nighttime insomnia and daytime sleepiness varying with the degree of coincidence between the internal circadian system and external clock time. At some times they will be appropriately matched with the outside time and will be sleeping fine, but eventually they will reach a point where their internal clocks are 180 degrees away from the actual day-night cycle, before gradually returning again to repeat another cycle. These predictable episodes of insomnia may recur indefinitely. The exact periodicity of the episodes depends on the intrinsic timing of the individual's circadian system, which in turn determines how much phase delay occurs each day. This type of recurrent insomnia is evident in the following case.

Walter, a 75-year-old married man, presented to the Sleep Disorders Center for help with recurrent insomnia. It had been a problem since shortly after World War II. During the war he was involved in combat while fighting in the Pacific campaign. He lost all vision, including light perception, as a result of a bomb explosion. He recovered well, except for the residual blindness. Ultimately, he started his own business, which became very successful. He continued to be involved with the business operations at the time of his evaluation. His complaint was episodic periods of insomnia and daytime sleepiness that seemed to last about two to three weeks and then would disappear for a few weeks. He and his wife noted that the episodes had been going on for most of their 50-year marriage and that the insomnia would appear and disappear for no apparent reason. Throughout the episodes he continued to follow his daytime work schedule; however, he found it more difficult to concentrate and remain awake. At night his sleep was very disrupted during the episodes. This included difficulty initiating and maintaining sleep. He presented for evaluation, since the effects of the insomnia had seemed more severe during the past few years. He was frustrated that he was less able to be involved with his business because of fatigue and sleepiness.

A graphic representation of this man's sleep-wake cycle during a 44-day period is shown in figure 3.2. The dark lines show the sleep hours on successive days derived from his sleep log. The graph is presented in a double plot format, which shows the successive 24-hour periods followed by the next day both to the right and below. This type of plot is useful to demonstrate trends over time. Clearly, in this case there is considerable variation in the timing and amount of sleep, and Walter's ability to achieve sufficient sleep during the nighttime is impaired. What is not represented here is the varying degree of daytime sleepiness that intruded on his attempts to remain productive throughout the day. His successful treatment included the nightly use of melatonin shortly before his bedtime. The melatonin was begun when his intrinsic cycle was at a phase when he was sleeping well at nighttime and feeling alert during the daytime. This helped to stabilize his circadian system to the 24-hour social rhythm.

Adequate total sleep, as well as full alertness during waking times, theoretically should be possible for these free-running blind individuals if they simply live their lives following their internal clocks: going to bed and getting up later each day without regard to the real-world clock time. At some point in their cycle, the bedtime would be 11:00 P.M.; however, several weeks later it would eventually become 11:00 A.M. before gradually returning several weeks later again to 11:00 P.M. For almost everyone, including the man in the case example, such a schedule would be highly impractical and inconvenient. The cause of this type of recurrent insomnia would remain a mystery without an appreciation of the slowly shifting circadian

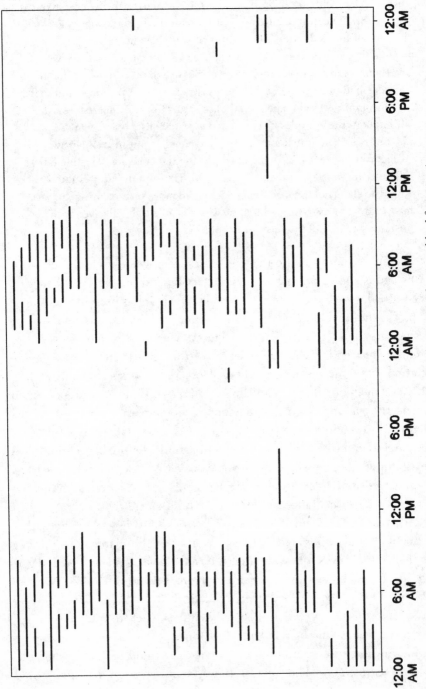

Figure 3.2 Double plot of sleep during successive days in a blind free-running case

sleepiness drive. The slowly changing pattern may hide the regularity of the cycle. This is in contrast to a rapidly shifting sleepiness pattern, as in the following example, which probably would become apparent quickly.

Forty-eight-Hour Cycle

We all are familiar with, to the point of taking for granted, the 24-hour cycle of sleepiness and arousal that usually results in our sleeping and wake time. It is odd, then, to encounter variations from the 24-hour periodicity. Rather dramatic are individuals whose cycling incorporates a major 48-hour component. There are several case reports of people with bipolar disorder who swing from depression to mania and back every other day, thus taking 48 hours for a full cycle (Wehr et al., 1982). They may be profoundly depressed one day and in an ecstatic or disorganized manic state the next day. Often with these patients there is a significant change in total sleep time on alternate nights: long sleep duration before depressed days and short sleep before manic days. The following is the case of a man who presented with very early awakening and high productivity alternating with longer sleep episodes and sluggishness throughout the day. In his case there was not a major mood component.

Samuel is a 60-year-old business executive presenting with a 4-year history of alternating nights of long and short sleep duration. There was no history of past or present psychiatric illness. His only current medication was levothyroxine for hypothyroidism, which was well controlled. Before the onset of this sleep difficulty, he had been quite satisfied with his nighttime sleep and daytime alertness. Generally, he had been sleeping from about 10:30 P.M. until about 6:30 A.M. He would nap only on very rare occasions. However, more recently he had been sleeping every other night from about 10:00 P.M. until a spontaneous awakening about 3:00 A.M. He would be fully alert at that time. He would get dressed and attend to a variety of projects before taking a long walk around dawn. He got to work early and enjoyed a highly productive day with full alertness. He never napped on these days. On the alternate nights, he still went to bed at about 10:00 P.M. but was still asleep when his wife's alarm awakened him at 6:30 A.M. He felt like remaining in bed but dragged himself into the shower. He felt rather sluggish. He drove to work, and some mornings he napped in his car before going into his office. He felt very unproductive on these days, and usually he kept his door shut so that he could nap intermittently and avoid social interactions. He felt much less productive and creative on these days. Since the pattern had been completely predictable, he had been able to schedule all important meetings and projects on the "good" days.

This man maintained a sleep log for several months. Figure 3.3 shows a double plot for a 30-day period. The alternation of his morning awakening time readily is evident in this graphic representation, as is the greater likelihood of napping on alternate days. An accurate prediction of the variation in the level of sleepiness and arousal during the day and night has been possible for this individual. Although the etiology of this 48-hour cycling is not entirely clear, it must be an internal clock–related phenomenon. Determining why the normal relationship of the homeostatic and circadian systems has been reorganized in such individuals ultimately may lead to a better understanding of the sleep-wake system in normal circumstances.

Homeostatic Breakdown

Most people are able to fall asleep at their bedtime because they have been awake all day or because the timing of their recent sleep and wakefulness has allowed a sufficient buildup of homeostatic sleep pressure. The circadian system helps organize the overall timing of sleep, and this generally helps prevent sleep from occurring randomly throughout the 24-hour day. The photoperiod and behavioral routines help reinforce the timing of the circadian sleep pattern. Circadian entrainment can be diminished in people who are significantly withdrawn and who avoid much variation in light exposure. It is possible for their sleep-wake cycles to become rather disorganized, with sleep occurring in multiple short episodes at any time of the day or night. They may never feel adequately refreshed and alert.

> Amy was a 32–year-old woman who lived with her parents. She had a long history of outpatient psychiatric treatment and had been given a wide variety of diagnoses, most recently panic disorder with agoraphobia. She was taking an antidepressant and a mood stabilizer. She had completed high school but dropped out of college after one year. She had limited employment in the past but had not worked for about 10 years. At the time of her evaluation in the Sleep Disorders Center, she rarely left her home, and mostly she stayed in her own room. She and her family

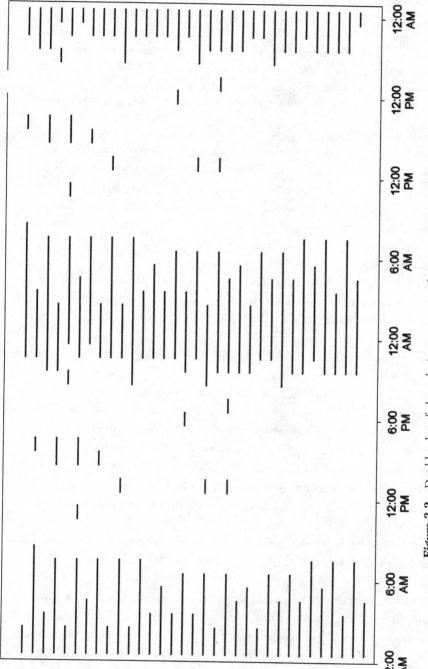

Figure 3.3 Double plot of sleep during successive days in a 48-hour sleep cycle

described her as having absolutely no regularity in a sleep-wake pattern. They said she was just as likely to be asleep during the daytime as at night-time. She never felt wide awake and energetic, nor did she ever feel that she had been deeply asleep. Usually, she was watching television or listening to music when she was awake, and rarely did she get much exercise. Her concerned parents wondered whether "fixing" her sleep problem would help solve the problem of her difficulty socializing and getting a job.

This patient's psychiatric symptoms strongly influenced her behavior, which in turn physiologically influenced her sleepiness-alertness pattern. All of this contributed to her downward spiral in social and occupational functioning. Behavioral changes, such as allowing appropriately timed exposure to bright light and darkness, as well as limiting her time in bed and increasing her physical activity, would be important steps in treatment. Of course, she still would need continued psychiatric therapy to improve her ability to leave the home comfortably.

Physical inactivity and limited variation in lightness and darkness may be relevant factors in the disorganized sleep-wake patterns identified in some institutionalized individuals, including some nursing home residents. Ancoli-Israel and Kripke (1989) showed that a sample group of nursing home patients studied at nighttime on the average were not asleep for more than one hour at a time, and during the daytime they were not awake for more than one hour at a time. Decreased activity and limited opportunities for circadian reinforcement through appropriately timed bright light and darkness may be relevant for some individuals living in institutions and perhaps also for some people experiencing depressive episodes associated with social withdrawal, isolation, and decreased motivation. They may spend excessive time in bed and have little exposure to bright light. The result may be that sleep never feels fully refreshing.

The Sleepiness-Arousal Balance and External Influences

Thus far, we have considered primarily aspects of the intrinsic circadian and homeostatic processes that can cause insomnia resulting from insufficient sleepiness at the desired time of sleep. A great variety of factors extrinsic to this primary sleep regulation also can influence the balance to varying degrees. This is especially troublesome when there is the promotion of a level of arousal that can overwhelm what might otherwise be an appropriate degree of sleepiness drive. That is, the homeostatic and circadian processes could be supplying adequate intrinsic sleepiness, but extrinsic arousing factors may result in an inability to sleep. Below are brief clinical vignettes of such situations of chronic sleep difficulty encountered in the Sleep Disorders Center among patients with complaints of insomnia.

- A 55-year-old woman awakens nightly at 3:00 A.M. to go to the bathroom. She worries about whether she will easily return to sleep, so, with hopes of relaxing, she smokes two cigarettes before getting back in bed. She then is frustrated that she lies in bed sleepless for the next two hours.
- A 28-year-old male weightlifter has problems getting to sleep at his bedtime. He decides to do a strenuous workout for one hour before his bedtime so that he will be "dead tired" and be able to fall asleep immediately. It is not successful.
- A 66-year-old woman has difficulty falling asleep most nights. She decides to eliminate the two cups of coffee she drinks each morning in hopes that this will help her fall asleep more easily. However, not considering potential stimulating effects, she continues to drink large amounts of iced tea throughout the afternoon and evening.
- A 42–year-old man frequently has difficulty with sleep onset. He sometimes experiences discomfort due to nasal congestion. He uses over-the-counter decongestants every night at bedtime. He is unaware that the medication has stimulating properties.
- A 48-year-old woman is frustrated with her nightly difficulty falling asleep. Although previously a rare drinker of alcoholic beverages, on the advice of friends she decides to try a glass of wine each night at bedtime. She falls asleep a little quicker but has more awakenings later during the night. She then tries two glasses of wine, but her sleep worsens due to more awakenings.
- A 35-year-old man has extended awakenings almost every night. He continues to work effectively but feels his concentration is poor. He and his primary care physician worry that depression may be causing the insomnia, so he begins taking an SSRI antidepressant. The sleep difficulty worsens.
- A 38-year-old woman had slept fine until three years previously, when a workplace injury resulted in multiple neck and back fractures. She

now experiences chronic pain, as well as difficulty falling asleep and frequent awakenings during the night.

- A 73-year-old woman has been treated for schizophrenia for several decades. She has chronic paranoid delusions about neighbors spying on her throughout the day and night. She is convinced that, when she is sleeping, they go through her important papers. She worries greatly every night at bedtime because of her fears that they will sneak into her apartment and possibly injure her.

- A 46-year-old man reports increasing sleep disruption during the previous two years. He has the sense of awakening dozens of times during the night for no apparent reason. He then returns to sleep quickly. He feels that his sleep no longer is refreshing and that his daytime performance is deteriorating. A sleep laboratory study is performed because of risk factors for sleep-disrupted breathing, and the results confirm a moderate degree of obstructive sleep apnea with frequent arousals. Treatment with nasal continuous positive airway pressure (CPAP) improves his sleep dramatically.

- A 54-year-old woman has had increasing difficulty falling asleep for about 10 years. When she gets in bed every night she experiences a very uncomfortable restlessness, mostly in her legs. Usually she needs to get out of bed and walk around for about 20 minutes before returning to bed and eventually falling asleep.

- A 38-year-old woman has had disrupted sleep since her late teens. Every night about one to two hours after falling asleep she will get out of bed and go to the kitchen to eat. Some nights this will be repeated one or two more times. Often she has no memory of the eating episodes, and she knows about them because of missing food, the presence of crumbs, or family members who witnessed her behavior. During the daytime she feels very fatigued.

- A 23-year-old woman slept well until six months before her evaluation. She had moved in with her boyfriend and found that her sleep was severely disrupted by his snoring. She feels fatigued throughout the daytime. She worries about their planned marriage and a sleepless future.

These examples represent the wide variety of processes that can interfere with the balance of sleepiness and arousal and that may promote difficulty initiating and maintaining sleep. In most of the cases, the described processes contribute to the alerting-arousal side of the balance and thereby overwhelm normal sleepiness levels. Some of these factors clearly are due to behavioral choices, such as late exercise and the use of caffeine, and some result from the arousing influence of other disorders that promote pain, discomfort, or restlessness.

Can sleepiness be increased further to counterbalance excessive arousal? This strategy, of course, is what is done commonly with the use of hypnotics and other sedating agents given with the intention of promoting sleep. This practice often is successful, but at times the arousal is too great or the baseline sleepiness too little to allow rapid induction of the onset of sleep.

The balance analogy of sleepiness and arousal should remain applicable in considering sleep disturbances generated by enduring personal vulnerabilities, stressful circumstances, and specific disease states. The circadian and homeostatic processes provide the sleepiness context for sleep to occur; however, many perturbations to the system are possible.

Of particular interest regarding circadian and homeostatic influences is the question of aging and the well-documented epidemiological evidence of worsened sleep among elderly individuals. One hypothesis is that insomnia in elderly persons is increased because of a blunted sleepiness drive resulting from a decreased amplitude in the circadian system; another argues that older individuals are less able to generate sufficient homeostatic sleep pressure to sustain consolidated nighttime sleep (Bliwise, 1993). These issues remain debatable. The topic of aging and sleep is revisited in chapter 7, under "Geriatric Insomnia."

Summary

Physiological and learning-reinforced drives influence the behavior of all animals, and with humans they may play important roles in clinical situations. Reasoning with this motivated behavior perspective is especially valuable when considering eating, sexual, and sleep disorders. The problem of insomnia can be approached using this perspective. The level of sleepiness one experiences is influenced strongly by the duration of prior wakefulness (homeostatic process) and the phase of the internal 24-hour rhythm (circadian process). Therefore, the likelihood of actually falling asleep when one attempts to do so is partly predictable from these processes. The converse also is true. Difficulty sleeping at a desired time, the complaint of insomnia, may be predictable and explainable solely with this model. Naturally, the identification of these underlying influences will have fundamental implications for treatment.

A balance analogy with opposite poles of sleepiness and arousal helps organize both intrinsic and extrinsic factors that promote normal and abnormal levels of sleepiness at any particular time. These factors include the homeostatic and circadian processes as well as a great variety of disorders, behaviors, emotional responses, and substance use.

A wide range of clinical presentations of insomnia is related directly to a predictably insufficient sleepiness drive. These include attempts to sleep without adequate homeostatic sleepiness, such as after an afternoon nap, as well as bedtimes out of synchronization with the circadian sleepiness cycle, typical of jet lag and rotating shift work schedules. This chapter has presented examples of real situations where people experience insomnia that is due primarily to problems related to the drive of sleepiness. The failure to identify and address these underlying influences may lead to chronic insomnia symptoms and possibly to ineffective treatment and other adverse sequelae. The identification and treatment of the circadian and/or homeostatic drive factors may be sufficient to solve the insomnia problem or, at least, can set the stage for treatment strategies associated with other perspectives.

4

The Dimensions of Sleep

Insomnia occurs in predisposed individuals because of their enduring vulnerabilities.

The Dimensional Perspective

Gradation and vulnerability are core concepts in the dimensional perspective. People vary along a wide assortment of dimensions. Height, blood
pressure, and serum potassium level are examples of easily measurable
physical characteristics, each with variation in a single dimension. In some
cases there is a normal or bell-shaped distribution of measured values in
the general population, and pathological processes may result in a skewed
distribution. Along some dimensional ranges, those individuals at one or
both extremes are at greater risk for developing particular problems than
are those in the middle ranges, who are more typical of the general population for that feature. Height is an enduring characteristic, while the vital
signs and laboratory values may show greater variation over time. Of primary interest here are those enduring individual features that may promote a longstanding vulnerability for various problems. In this regard,
McHugh and Slavney (1998) describe a paradigm where a *potential*
exposed to a *provocation* results in a *response*. Consider tallness: extraordinary height is only a potential problem until the provocation of a short
doorway reveals the increased risk of a head-banging response.

Although particular features may be measurable along defined scales,
threshold values may be posited to separate a range into categories. For
example, with serum potassium one can define value bins with descriptors
such as dangerously low, low, normal, high, and dangerously high. We
think of the dangerously low and high portions of the range as increasing

the risk of arrhythmia and, perhaps, death. The vital sign extremes of excessively low or high blood pressure, heart rate, and body temperature obviously also are associated with severe and potentially life-threatening vulnerabilities. Although the defined categories may be important and certainly convenient, often the absolute breakpoint values are somewhat arbitrary and not directly predictive of particular responses. The difference between normal and abnormal may be a very fine line or a wide frontier. Accordingly, caution is necessary in defining the breakpoints. The categorical trees should not obscure the dimensional forest.

Often physical dimensions are obvious and easy to measure, and even those that involve challenging measurements tend not to be conceptually ambiguous. Although less directly observable, certain features in mental life also may be formulated in dimensional terms. For instance, the field of psychometrics rests on a dimensional foundation. McHugh and Slavney offer intelligence as an excellent example of a formulated dimension in the cognitive arena. Intelligence, as indicated by psychometric instruments, represents an innate potential that is revealed by life circumstances. Lower intelligence correlates with a decreased ability to cope with challenging situations, such as ones that demand abstract reasoning. The lower the intelligence score, the higher the vulnerability.

Characteristics of personality often are conceived in terms of variation within a population. Individuals are seen as exhibiting greater or lesser degrees of particular personality features, which ultimately are defined in terms of potentials—that is, generally predicting how one might respond emotionally or behaviorally in various circumstances (provocations). This broad personality realm encompasses an individual's temperament or affective disposition. These enduring characteristics are viewed as constitutional proclivities, which at more extreme degrees increase the vulnerability for clinical problems. Once again, it is the combination of this latent vulnerability and the degree of circumstantial stress that contributes to the response, which might include clinically significant symptoms.

The dimensionality of personality characteristics is readily apparent in the multitude of instruments that have been developed to assess personality. These may indicate the degree to which an individual exhibits features such as emotional stability, introversion and extraversion, openness, agreeableness, conscientiousness, various aptitudes and attitudes, and hundreds of other personality constructs. The personality tests may be oriented to normal features, as with the NEO Personality Inventory, or to psychopathological assessment. Some of these instruments, such as the Minnesota Multiphasic Personality Inventory (MMPI), may use constellations of dimensional scores in assessing a person. Dimensional reasoning in psychiatry has broad applications in clinical situations. In theory, at least, the *Diagnostic and Statistical Manual of Mental Disorders* (DSM-IV) axis II diagnoses are based on this premise of the dimensional variation in personality characteristics. Those individuals formally diagnosed with personality disorders have reached a certain threshold of symptoms or historical features at which their enduring personality characteristics are seen as contributing to a variety of possible life problems.

The question to be addressed here is to what extent the problems of insomnia sufferers can be illuminated by a consideration of how people may vary along one or more continua. What intrinsic characteristics increase one's vulnerability for inadequate sleep? Are there scales where scores in a particular range predict insomnia complaints? Two major directions for exploring these issues are by measuring aspects of sleep and related rhythms and by assessing personality characteristics. In both of these areas, dimensional reasoning has been implicit in explanatory models of sleep disturbances involving insomnia as a primary complaint.

The Dimensions of Sleep

In the investigation of sleep, as in all scientific inquiry, observation and measurement allow the interrelated processes of identification and creation of dimensions: phenomena are observed and described, and scales with defined increments are constructed. The realm of sleep and wakefulness includes a variety of potential spectra. Long before modern technological advances, the sleep-wake dichotomy had been self-evident, along with a general sense of "how deeply asleep" and "how much awake" one might be. Early scientific studies of sleep observed its depth and described its relation to such features as physical movements, breathing patterns, and arousability. The duration of observed sleep easily could be measured. Then, beginning in the 1920s with the advent of the electroencephalogram (EEG), a multitude of signal-derived features of sleep and wakefulness could be monitored.

A basic spectrum of sleep is the simple duration, whether it is derived from subjective report or objective measurement. We have seen that sleep length and timing are influenced primarily by the homeostatic and circadian processes and that about eight hours really does represent the typical average sleep need. However, there does seem to be a spectrum ranging from those who need less to those who need more sleep for optimal functioning. Clearly, the vast majority of individuals in our society averaging less than about seven hours of sleep per night do so by external schedule constraints directly influencing the time available for sleep. The consequences of insufficient sleep for this group are measurable in various waking parameters, as noted in chapter 2. However, a small percentage of people do seem to accomplish their sleep need in a relatively short time. These so-called short sleepers will awaken spontaneously after perhaps six hours or less and will demonstrate evidence of full alertness throughout the waking hours. There are reports of extreme short sleepers averaging less than four hours nightly; however, these are quite rare and are not well studied or documented.

The natural and unimpaired short sleepers occupy one end of the sleep duration spectrum along with many chronically insomniac persons, who find their condition unnatural and impairing. Of course, the difference is clear: the latter complain. While relatively short nighttime sleep without adverse daytime consequences may be viewed as a blessing, allowing someone more hours of wakefulness to enjoy and to use productively, some people, as evidenced in the case below, worry that this proclivity may represent an underlying problem.

> *The Short Sleeper:* George was a 32–year-old, midlevel manager with a large investment firm. He was married and had two small children. He had developed a typical routine of spending time with his family in the early evening, and after the children went to bed around 8:00 P.M. he turned to his computer for various projects related to his work and personal finances. He would begin to feel somewhat sleepy by about 11:00 P.M., and he almost always was asleep by midnight. He and his wife concurred that he seemed to sleep soundly during the night. His concern prompting evaluation in the Sleep Disorders Center was that he never could sleep past 5:00 A.M., and often his spontaneous awakening was closer to 4:30 A.M. Everyone else in the house slept another two hours in the morning. He worried that he might have a sleep disorder that prevented further sleep. His history included no evidence of daytime sleepiness, impairment, or distress. He never was tempted to nap, and he felt fully productive throughout the daytime.

As a short sleeper, this man worried that he had insomnia, but, in actuality, he simply was not suffering at all. His being at the short end of the duration spectrum raised the question of abnormality. Similar concerns may occur at the opposite end of the spectrum. People with unusually long sleep requirements may be worried that a fundamental inadequacy in their sleep leads them to be excessively sleepy. So-called long sleepers, who may require an average of nine hours or more per night to prevent symptoms of insufficient sleep, often complain about their inconvenient need to sleep so much or about the daytime sleepiness they experience when they get only eight hours of sleep at night. They may argue that, since they are sleeping the officially recommended amount (eight hours), there must be something fundamentally inadequate about the sleep they achieve and that this may be a manifestation of insomnia.

> *The Long Sleeper*: Madelyn was a 45-year-old woman who had been working as a secretary for about 20 years. She was married and had two teenage children. She complained of chronic sleepiness for "as long as I can remember." She felt as though she needed at least 10 hours of sleep to feel awake the next day, but this occurred only during vacations. Typically, she was rather sleepy by 8:00 P.M., and she managed to get to bed and fall asleep quickly by 10:00 P.M. She felt that she slept "like a log," and she had to drag herself out of bed after the 6:00 A.M. alarm to get the day going for herself and her family. Eventually, she complained to her primary care physician that there must be something wrong with her sleep, since she never seemed to be able to get enough of it. Her history did not include features suggestive of primary disorders known to promote hypersomnolence.

Knowing that insomnia may cause daytime sleepiness and poor concentration, Madelyn figured that she must have it. By history, however, it seems more likely that her enduring vulnerability was her constitutional need for a greater than average amount of sleep. Her relatively high sleep requirement was not matched by her schedule, which allotted only what seemed to be the normal amount, that is, eight hours.

Aside from the total duration, sleep also may be examined in terms of its constituent elements identifiable from the EEG signal and other physiological monitoring. Current sleep stage conventions, developed in the 1960s, divide sleep into rapid eye movement (REM) and non-REM (NREM), which is divided further into four stages of increasing depth.

Studies have established age-related normal ranges for these stages in terms of total amounts (usually in minutes per stage) and percentages of total nighttime sleep. Are there enduring tendencies for someone to fall at high, average, or low total amounts or percentages of these sleep stages, which ultimately could promote the insomnia experience? It certainly is true that major changes in sleep architecture may correspond with the experience of insomnia due to various underlying processes. For instance, during an episode of insomnia, sleep may be lighter, as evidenced by relatively high amounts of NREM stage 1 sleep or relatively low amounts of NREM stages 3 and 4. Sleep may be so disrupted that normal REM activity cannot be sustained and, therefore, the REM amount and percentage are decreased. However, these abnormalities of sleep architecture probably are integral to the insomnia process, as opposed to predisposing the person to the sleepless experience. Whatever is disrupting the sleep may be influencing the architecture as well as the subjective experience. Presently, there is no clear evidence that an antecedent alteration of sleep stages increases the vulnerability to insomnia.

In addition to describing sleep with the traditional model of a sleep stage label attached to each 30-second epoch to create a hypnogram, it is possible to analyze the EEG signal to determine the activity in different frequency ranges. For example, the relative power of delta, theta, alpha, beta, or any other defined frequency bin can be examined throughout a sleep period (see table 2.1). Composite or longitudinal values can be examined and compared. There may be low delta activity and high alpha, beta, and even gamma activity associated with the light sleep of insomnia. These dimensional comparisons ultimately may play an important role in establishing a relationship between the EEG signal and the sleep-wake experience. The one clinical situation where a frequency excess could be viewed as increasing the vulnerability for insomnia is with fibromyalgia. Many individuals diagnosed with this disorder experience symptoms of chronic insomnia. Patients with fibromyalgia tend to have excessive amounts of alpha activity, which under normal circumstances is associated with the relaxed waking state (Moldofsky et al., 1975). Perhaps excess in this dimension of wake-related EEG activity occurring during sleep negatively influences the perception of sleep.

Chronic Fatigue: Karen was a 45-year-old woman who complained of persistent daytime fatigue of about six years duration, having begun after an episode of mononucleosis. Previously, she had worked full time, but three years before her evaluation in the Sleep Disorders Center she was diagnosed with fibromyalgia, and she received disability payments because of her severe fatigue symptoms. She found that the fatigue markedly impaired her ability to perform even minimal household chores. Although sleepy during the daytime, she would avoid napping. Typically, she would get in bed and attempt to sleep at about 9:00 P.M.; however, usually it would take her several hours to fall sleep. She described a great craving for sleep but a sense that her mind and body prevented it. After eventually falling asleep, she would experience multiple awakenings and usually have difficulty returning to sleep. Most days she was out of bed for the day about 9:00 A.M. but sometimes rose as late as 11:00 A.M. She avoided all caffeine and alcohol. She was on no prescribed medication, although she regularly took a variety of herbal substances. She was hopeful that an underlying sleep disorder would be identified and treated, so that she again could be active and energetic during the daytime.

Another common sleep measurement resulting in a dimension with some relevance to insomnia is the degree of daytime sleepiness indicated by the Multiple Sleep Latency Test (MSLT) (see chap. 3). A shorter average latency to sleep onset during the four to five daytime naps suggests greater sleepiness. However, as noted in chapter 1, only some people complaining of insufficient nighttime sleep experience a compensatory increase in sleepiness during the daytime. Therefore, the correlation between the insomnia complaint and the daytime sleepiness dimension is not strong. It is unlikely that this dimension of daytime sleepiness directly increases the vulnerability for insomnia.

The most powerful evidence of dimensional influence on the development of insomnia symptoms is manifest in the circadian rhythm disorders, primarily the advanced and delayed sleep phase syndromes (Campbell et al., 1999). These two disorders and the altered circadian timing influence in subsyndromal cases contribute to the sleep disturbance in a surprisingly large percentage of people suffering with insomnia. Since the circadian system significantly regulates the timing of sleep under normal circumstances, it is easy to see that abnormal circadian timing causes abnormal times of sleepiness and arousal. If the desired time for sleep corresponds with the circadian wakeful phase, then sleeplessness may result.

The circadian system helps promote a sleep period from about 10:00 or 11:00 P.M. until 6:00 or 7:00 A.M. for most individuals, but in the general population there is a spectrum in the intrinsic rhythm, with a range from the advanced-type "early birds" to the delayed-type "night owls." Many people live quite successfully with an "early to bed, early to rise" pattern or, conversely, habitually stay up fairly late and then sleep late the next day. However, others suffer considerably because of the mismatch between their internal circadian sleep promotion and their desired sleep time or the requirements of their schedule. This important enduring vulnerability often is overlooked as a cause of chronic sleep disturbance.

The intrinsic timing of the circadian system seems to be relatively stable, and it generally incorporates a developmental trend. Young children often sleep 9 to 10 hours from the mid-evening until shortly after dawn, but with puberty there commonly is a delay, resulting in a later arrival of sleepiness and a corresponding continued expression of sleepiness into the morning daylight hours. The result, of course, is going to bed later and, whenever circumstances allow, sleeping later the next day. With transition into adulthood, most people gradually shift back to an earlier sleep and wake time, and the process continues such that many elderly people go to bed and awaken even earlier than they had throughout much of their adult lives. Although this moderate trend applies to the majority of the population, some people experience dramatic extremes, and some will persist at various degrees of severity at either end of this sleep-wake timing spectrum. There now is evidence that some individuals have an advanced sleep phase pattern due to a familial circadian rhythm variant (Jones et al., 1999).

The extent to which this sleep-timing tendency represents a dimension is highlighted with the Morningness-Eveningness Scale developed by Horne and Ostberg (1976). This is a self-completed questionnaire focusing on behaviors and preferences for performing various activities at different hours of the day. Points accumulated from the 19 questions range from 16 to 86. The distribution is divided into categories of definitely morning type, moderately morning type, neither type, moderately evening type, and definitely evening type. Generally, older individuals are more likely to fall into the morning types and younger people (adolescents and young adults) into the evening types; however, there are some older severe evening types and younger severe morning types.

A relatively early evening sleepiness and a spontaneous early-morning awakening characterize the advanced sleep pattern, typical of the morning types on the Morningness-Eveningness Scale. For some people, the advance will have been to a mild degree and even been highly effective in their lifestyle for many years but then exacerbate to a more moderate or severe early timing. If those with this tendency go to bed and fall asleep very early, they should have the opportunity for sufficient sleep, thereby allowing them appropriate daytime alertness. However, their intrinsically promoted sleep hours may be 8:00 P.M. to 4:00 A.M., and this may not be consistent with work and family requirements or with social or leisure desires. Of course, people with this advanced pattern often do not go to bed that early. Usually, they remain active in the evening in spite of increasing sleepiness, and eventually they go to bed and fall asleep quite rapidly. Although they have been awake later in the evening, generally they do not sleep correspondingly later the following morning. Most will report that they wake up too early no matter what time they go to bed. The intrinsic circadian arousing influence causes either a full awakening with no return to sleep or extremely light and interrupted sleep during the last few hours of the night. Since this is a persistent tendency, chronic sleep insufficiency with subsequent daytime fatigue and sleepiness often ensues. This combination of daytime impairment and a complaint of early-morning awakening commonly is the presenting history in people with this syndrome.

The Older Early Bird: Rose was a 66-year-old woman who lived alone in a condominium. She had long been employed full time in customer relations, and she was active socially and pursued various cultural and leisure interests. She was in good health. Her psychiatric history did include three episodes of major depression requiring hospitalization; however, the most recent had been more than 30 years ago. Generally, she felt that her mood had been good in recent years. She presented to the Sleep Disorders Center with a complaint of persistent early-morning awakening for almost 20 years. She had tried many different antidepressants and hypnotics without great success, and most recently she had been taking clonazepam and gabapentin. Generally, she was sleepy in the early to mid-evening. She would go to bed by 10:30 P.M. and fall asleep instantly. She would sleep soundly until about 3:00 A.M. Often she was unable to return to sleep again, or, if she did, her sleep seemed very light. She never used an alarm clock. She would get out of bed for the day by 7:00 A.M. She felt fatigued throughout the day, but she avoided napping. She reported that she had read various books on sleep problems and had tried to follow what seemed to be appropriate advice on sleep hygiene. In the attempt to promote relaxation and deeper sleep, she kept her home very dark in the evening. She usually used candlelight only, and she would wear sunglasses while watching television in the evening. She had read that dawn light was good to stabilize the sleep-wake cycle, so she would open all the curtains immediately when she got out of bed in the morning.

Rose shares with many older individuals a persistent and very frustrating pattern of early-morning awakening that has been resistant to various attempted treatment strategies. Rose followed general sleep hygiene advice that seemed to make sense; in actuality, however, it was having the exact opposite effect from what she had desired. Her purposeful dim light evenings and bright light mornings were reinforcing her already too advanced circadian system. Her multiple previous treatment strategies had missed this key underlying influence. Ultimately, strategic exposure to bright light and darkness played a major therapeutic role for her. Light-related strategies are explored further in chapter 7.

The degree to which the circadian influence on sleep timing represents a clinical problem is largely relative. The advanced sleep tendency may be a heavenly match for the person living a monastic existence and arising for 4:00 A.M. prayers. It may be disastrous for another person who is required to work late in the evening. A circadian mismatch between husband and wife can lead directly to significant marital discord. Along the spectrum from mild to severe, those individuals who experience significant problems due to this enduring circadian vulnerability may meet criteria for the formal *International Classification of Sleep Disorders Diagnostic and Coding Manual* (ICSD) diagnosis of advanced sleep phase syndrome. A relatively young person with the disorder is represented in the following case.

The Younger Early Bird: Joyce was a 27-year-old, single woman who lived alone. She worked full time as an attorney. She noted that she had always tended to be an "early bird" and that she had never needed to use an alarm clock. She came to the Sleep Disorders Center because of her inability to get sufficient sleep at night and her subsequent fatigue and sleepiness during the daytime. She felt that she could not think clearly and was not very productive during the daytime. She never napped and did not experience inadvertent sleep episodes. She often had some difficulty falling asleep; however, she always awoke quite early. She would become very sleepy early in the evening, and typically she would go to bed between 8:30 P.M. and 9:00 P.M. From past experience she knew that if she stayed up later she still would not sleep later the next day and that she would feel even worse that day. On a good night she might sleep until 4:30 A.M., but often she would awaken spontaneously well before that time. She was always out of bed early, and usually she was at work by

7:30 A.M. She enjoyed a variety of outdoor activities during the daytime; however, she severely restricted evening social activities because of her sleepiness at that time and because of the price she felt she would pay the following day. She had tried an assortment of herbal preparations, as well as over-the-counter (OTC) and prescription hypnotic agents, all with rather limited success.

It is clear that profound social implications resulted from Joyce's circadian phase predisposition. One reason that the advanced sleep pattern often is not identified is that usually it does not directly interfere with work and school, except in circumstances of chronic sleep insufficiency and subsequent daytime impairment. Too often, people presenting with early-morning awakening automatically have been assumed to have a depressive disorder, which was thought to be the primary cause of the sleep disturbance. Certainly, mood disorders have a high priority in the differential diagnosis of this condition; however, depression-related early-morning awakening is likely to be more episodic, in contrast to the relatively persistent advanced sleep phase tendency due to the intrinsic circadian system. Accordingly, antidepressants are not likely to be helpful for the circadian phase advance. Neither have hypnotics typically been beneficial, as these are most efficacious in promoting sleep during the first several hours after a bedtime dose. The annoying early-morning awakening usually is just a few hours before the desired awakening, and it is too late then to use the hypnotic. Joyce was able to sleep later in the morning after she initiated therapeutic exposure to bright light in the evening and avoided light around dawn.

One curious feature of these circadian morning types is the frequent difficulty they encounter with schedule changes, such as those occurring with shifts in work schedule and jet lag. Overall, they seem to have less flexibility with these time shifts. This relative intolerance results in more severe and prolonged symptoms. This is in contrast to those at the other extreme of the circadian phase spectrum, who typically have less difficulty with schedule changes.

Those described as "night owls" or evening types, thus having a delayed sleep phase pattern, occupy the opposite end of this circadian sleep-time-propensity dimension. They find it easy to stay up late and sleep late the following day. Some of them thrive on the productivity, social activities, solitude, or leisure pursuits (e.g., late-night television, reading, internet surfing) they are able to enjoy during the late evening and early morning hours. The ability then to sleep until the late morning or even into the afternoon affords them sufficient total sleep and, consequently, optimum alertness during their waking hours. They may gravitate toward flexible work hours allowing a relatively late arrival or to permanent schedules on evening and night shifts. This delayed sleep phase tendency is quite common to a mild or moderate degree among people in their mid- to later teens and among many in their 20s. Some people will persist with this tendency throughout adulthood, and some cases remain apparent in geriatric populations.

Although some individuals with this delayed circadian proclivity have adapted their lives successfully to their biological predisposition, for many there is a significant vulnerability for sleep-wake cycle disturbance whenever they attempt to follow an otherwise normal schedule. Obviously, many do not have the luxury to sleep whenever they feel like it; people's schedules often are not entirely under their control. There may be a longstanding internal-external schedule mismatch (e.g., military service). For these individuals there is chronic difficulty falling asleep at a customary bedtime and difficulty getting up at an appropriate time in the morning. In extreme circumstances they will be diagnosable with the ICSD designation delayed sleep phase syndrome.

Although the advanced sleep phase pattern mostly is a great annoyance and inconvenience, the delayed pattern has greater potential to interfere considerably with one's educational and occupational functioning. There are two common and frequently overlapping chief complaints: chronic sleep-onset insomnia and chronic difficulty awakening at a desired early-morning hour. Excessive daytime sleepiness also is a common accompaniment. Those afflicted with this syndrome are sleepy in the morning due to circadian phase delay, and often they are sleepy later in the day due to chronic sleep insufficiency resulting from curtailed sleep in the morning. In severe cases, patients may present because of failing performance at school or repeated job loss from chronic tardiness. For this syndrome, misdiagnosis and inappropriate treatment are very common.

Persons with delayed sleep phase syndrome typically have attempted various failed strategies to promote falling asleep at a desired earlier time. Either they attempt sleep at the earlier time and remain sleepless and frustrated in bed for hours before eventually falling asleep, or they realize that an earlier sleep onset is impossible and do not bother to go to bed until rather late. Typical relaxation and behavioral techniques fail because sleepiness is absent simply because of the underlying circadian delay. In fact, the desired bedtime may be in these delayed individuals' circadian zone of minimum sleepiness, which for normally phased sleepers would be at some point around 7:00 P.M. to 9:00 P.M. Even hypnotic and other sedating medications often are of limited benefit in promoting a rapid sleep onset for phase-delayed patients who take them at an early desired bedtime; these patients experience minimum intrinsic sleepiness at that hour.

Once those individuals with the delayed sleep phase pattern do fall asleep, generally they can remain asleep for a normal length of time, as long as there are no external interruptions. If they have been asleep only a few hours and are in their delayed circadian zone of maximum sleepiness, an external interruption (e.g., alarm clock) might need to be of a relatively great magnitude to produce a sustained awakening. The measures undertaken in the attempt to guarantee an on-time awakening may be very impressive, matching the profound sleepiness and, at least for that moment, the intense desire to remain in bed sleeping. For severely delayed sleepers at 8:00 A.M., nothing else may matter except further immediate sleep. What might have been viewed as extremely important the night before, such as getting to a morning college course exam or avoiding another confrontation with the boss about chronic tardiness, lessens considerably to the point of no longer achieving sufficient importance to warrant getting out of bed. Concern for consequences may evaporate temporarily. Shame and embarrassment may follow eventually but usually too late. These severely delayed sleepers often tell of using multiple alarm clocks (sometimes attached to loud stereo systems), arranging for friends or family to telephone them repeatedly, or having other household members force them out of bed. Once fully awake, they still may need to contend with excessive sleepiness later in the day. Since they are at risk for chronic sleep insufficiency, they may fall asleep during daytime activities, especially during morning lectures or meetings and, in severe cases, while driving or operating equipment.

In most cases of delayed sleep phase, the individuals are able to identify the onset of the tendency in the teen years. A common history is for people to report that, while in high school, they frequently slept late during weekends and vacations but managed to get up and function appropriately on school days. However, soon after beginning college, especially if living in a dormitory, they fell into a chronic pattern of staying up rather late studying and socializing and then sleeping late into the morning. They quickly began to avoid, whenever possible, early or midmorning classes.

Problems arose whenever they needed to be up early, perhaps for a required early class. Sometimes, to be sure that they would be up for an 8:00 A.M. exam, they would simply stay up all night, knowing that this was their best guarantee for getting there. Common in the history also is the attempt to sustain daytime morning sleep as late as possible by blocking out outside light. This combination of the intrinsic rhythm and behaviors influencing rhythm reinforcement contributes to the intractable problem.

Two specific questions, especially in this younger population, may reveal answers that, if not pathognomonic for the condition, at least may offer interesting supportive evidence. The first inquiry is, "Do you have much light coming into your bedroom window?" Although there are exceptions, most will reply immediately that they hate the morning light, and many will tell of having installed blackout curtains or other creative solutions to their perceived problem with morning light. One student said that he had the nickname of Dracula because of his reputation for being active throughout the night and his purposeful avoidance of morning light. The following case epitomizes the avoidance of morning light in phase-delayed individuals.

> *College Dorm Phase Delay:* Michael was an 18-year-old student in his first year of college. He lived in a dormitory except on weekends, when he slept in his bedroom at his parent's home nearby. During the previous few years, he had found it very easy to stay up late and then sleep well into the following daytime. This tendency was a mild problem during his last year of high school; however, in college it had worsened dramatically. If he tried to go to sleep relatively early, which for him was about midnight, he would remain sleepless for several hours. Usually, he would do schoolwork late at night and go to bed around 2:00 or 3:00 A.M., and sometimes he would simply stay up the entire night and the following day. Typically, he would be asleep by 4:00 or 5:00 A.M., and then he would sleep soundly for several hours. Many days he would get up at 10:00 A.M., although it was not uncommon for him to sleep well into the afternoon or even to the early evening. Often during the daytime he felt rather sleepy and experienced poor concentration. He said that he felt like a "zombie," especially in the morning. He felt that his inability to get enough sleep at night was affecting his performance at school significantly. He had tried relaxation techniques and OTC hypnotics with no benefit. In the attempt to get as much sleep as possible during the daytime, he kept his bedroom in his parents' home extremely dark with blackout curtains. In his dormitory room he had placed his mattress on the

floor and turned the bed frame upside down such that it was raised several feet above the mattress. Heavy covers were draped around the side, blocking out the light and effectively creating a dark cave for his sleeping environment. He kept a fan running for ventilation and had altered the thermostat to keep the room rather cold.

Clearly, this young man's behavior of blocking out the daylight had a deleterious permissive effect of allowing further delay in his circadian system, and ultimately it contributed to his worsening academic difficulties. While the darkness during the morning daylight hours helped him make up for lost nighttime sleep, it denied him the primary entraining influence that might be beneficial in helping to shift his circadian system earlier. By way of nature he had the constitutional vulnerability for a delayed sleep-wake cycle; however, he had nurtured this potential much further through behavioral choices.

The other valuable question for the phase-delayed college student is, "How much time do you need from the alarm clock going off until when you need to be in class?" A precise answer, especially a short duration, highlights that this has been an important issue for the individual. This concern for trying to sleep until the very last minute is evident in the following case.

> **The Campus Racer:** Jennifer was a 19-year-old woman in her second year of college and living in a dormitory. In addition to a full academic schedule, she also worked part time in a retail setting. She regarded herself as a "night owl," as she always stayed up rather late and slept late into the following day. Her part-time employment was in the evening, and she never scheduled herself for classes before 10:00 A.M. or, preferably, 11:00 A.M. She presented to the Sleep Disorders Center because of her frustration at not being able to fall asleep until about 3:00 A.M. and her extreme difficulty awakening in the morning. She often had been late for classes, but through organizing herself as much as possible the night before, she could be in class only 18 minutes after her alarm clock awakened her.

Many of these young phase-delayed individuals survive by doing schoolwork during their peak alertness at nighttime and by making as many preparations as possible for the following day before going to bed. For morning classes they will dress very quickly, groom minimally, waste no time eating, and perhaps return for a nap afterward. One male student described wearing a baseball cap to his first class so that he would not have to spend extra time combing his hair.

Aside from the deterioration between high school and college, a less common but still occasionally identifiable transition point for the marked worsening of phase-delay symptoms is retirement. Some people with the underlying tendency to phase delay have managed decades of stable employment with an early-morning schedule only to find that, without the constant reinforcing influence of early awakening and dawn light exposure, the sleep-wake cycle delays dramatically. Instead of falling asleep regularly at 11:00 P.M., now it is 4:00 A.M., and instead of getting up at 7:00 A.M., now it is noon. In some cases, the severe and intractable sleep-wake timing delay begins after travel, vacations, or temporary changes in work schedule.

> *Retirement Phase Delay:* Lila, a 74-year-old woman, presented to the Sleep Disorders Center because of her great concerns about her sleep-wake cycle. Generally, she had slept well through most of her life until gradually she was staying up later and sleeping later the following day. Ultimately, she found that she was unable to sleep at an earlier desired bedtime, so she gave up and simply followed what seemed to her an uncontrollable sleep tendency. Once she fell asleep, she was able to remain asleep, and she found that she attained sufficient sleep by sleeping rather late into the daytime. In fact, it was her concern about sleeping too much that eventually prompted her evaluation. The tendency to go to bed later and later began with her husband's retirement. At that time he began staying up later, so they drifted to later bedtimes together. After several years, they routinely were going to bed around dawn and awakening in the midafternoon. This pattern was a minor nuisance for them, as they missed opportunities for various daytime activities and there was no way to socialize with others during their wakeful hours throughout the night. What finally greatly distressed Lila was the phenomenon she termed "sleeping through," whereby she would not awaken in the afternoon but would continue sleeping until the following morning. She might get up for a bathroom visit, but she remained quite sleepy and immediately returned to sleep again without engaging in any other activities. These extended sleep episodes had been occurring approximately once per week. This excessive sleeping interfered with her daily schedule for antihypertensive medication. She also felt that she was sleeping her life away. Most recently, her major concern was about her husband, who had developed mild symptoms of dementia and was unsupervised during her uncontrollable sleeping.

Lila's normal sleep-wake cycle throughout most of her life was influenced by her husband's schedule. As he slept later, she no longer felt compelled to get up early. Together they drifted later and later. She then progressed to the more serious problem of "sleeping through" and missing an entire day. This tendency to experience these ultralong-duration sleep episodes seems to be a rather malignant complication of the most severe cases of delayed sleep phase syndrome. The severely delayed pattern may undermine light entrainment during the appropriate phase of the circadian cycle. Several other patients, with a wide range of ages, have presented to the Sleep Disorders Center with similar histories of progressive phase delay eventually evolving into frequent episodes of sleeping through their usual waking periods. All were quite distressed about both the uncontrollable nature of the extended sleep episodes and the inability to attend to necessary activities.

People with a severely delayed sleep phase pattern that causes clear life problems rarely receive much sympathy or understanding regarding this vulnerability. They are more likely to be told that they are lazy and unmotivated. They hear, "Just go to bed earlier" or "Just get up earlier." They may be regarded as poor students or poor employees. Those without this problem often are unable to relate to the difficulty experienced by these patients. Many afflicted individuals feel quite frustrated and helpless about this pervasive problem. Although motivation may evaporate at the phase of profound sleepiness, generally they are motivated to try anything that might help them better control their lives.

If the photoperiod effectively entrains most humans to nighttime sleep and spontaneous awakenings at or soon after dawn, why is it that some people find themselves entrenched in undesirable sleep-time predispositions that are much earlier or much later than those of most people? To date there is no fully adequate explanation; however, theoretical speculation has focused on the ability of light to promote entrainment at different portions of the phase-response curve and on genetically determined abnormalities of the molecular circadian clock.

The recognition of these circadian rhythm disorders requires an appreciation of the primary clinical characteristics, particularly the longstanding vulnerability and the developmental trends. The influence of the advanced and delayed circadian tendencies clearly relates to the 24-hour cycle. Therefore, in evaluating an individual presenting with insomnia symptoms, it is important to focus not just on the time of sleeplessness but also on the entire daily pattern of sleepiness and alertness, as well as on how it has evolved longitudinally. The insomnia of the circadian rhythm disorders is part of a predictable rhythm.

Personality and Sleep

Are there enduring characteristics in the realm of personality, particularly aspects of temperament, which increase a person's vulnerability to experiencing insomnia? If these dispositional features are dimensionally conceived, is it possible to suggest that the risk of insomnia increases for those individuals at one or both dimensional extremes? Such dimensional reasoning has been at the foundation of some explanatory models of insomnia. Paradigms of this type potentially are valuable in identifying causative factors and in suggesting psychotherapeutic strategies for insomnia sufferers.

Anthony and Joyce Kales (1984) have been major proponents of the association between psychological predisposition and chronic insomnia. In studying chronic insomnia populations and controls, employing psychiatric evaluations and various psychological measurement instruments, they conclude that some degree of psychopathology always is present with persistent insomnia. They suggest that the "findings of lifelong emotional difficulties preceding chronic insomnia may explain why episodes of stress-induced sleeplessness are transient for most people, while for others they become an ingrained pattern" (Kales and Kales, 1984, p. 113). In one study of one hundred persons with chronic insomnia, 100 percent of them were diagnosed with DSM-III axis I and/or axis II disorders.

Discussions in the literature on sleep disorders regarding personality and insomnia often center on the idea of internalization. It is argued that people who tend to internalize their emotions, thereby not expressing their feelings and emotional conflicts, are at increased risk for the development of chronic insomnia. Accordingly, populations suffering from chronic insomnia should have a greater percentage of internalizers than do populations of matched controls. Furthermore, populations of internalizers should contain more insomniac persons than do noninternalizer groups. The challenge, of course, is validly representing the internalization construct to identify who is high and who is low for this feature.

Kales and Kales (1984) evaluated several hundred chronically insomniac persons and controls with the MMPI and reported significant scale elevations and psychopathology suggested by code patterns. The highest scale elevations for the insomnia group were depression, psychasthenia, and conversion hysteria. The majority of the chronic insomniac persons showed elevations consistent with "pessimistic thinking, inhibition of anger, self-depreciation, and persistent worrying" (p. 115). Generally, Kales and Kales found that, throughout the insomnia age spectrum, the MMPI scores indicated "neurotic depression, apprehension, inhibition, rumination, and an inability to outwardly discharge anger" (p. 118).

From their research on groups of chronic insomnia sufferers, Kales and Kales developed an internalization hypothesis of the cause of chronic insomnia. They proposed that the internalization of psychological disturbance, as evidenced by the MMPI results, leads to chronic insomnia because the unresolved and internalized conflicts result in emotional arousal and subsequently create physiological activation. This aroused state occurs both before and during sleep. With the emergence of insomnia comes apprehension about continued sleep difficulty and, ultimately, an excessive focus on and worry about sleep that lead to further insomnia. Eventually, the fear of not sleeping may provoke sufficient emotional distress to fuel persistent physiological activation. Finally, a conditioned pattern of chronic insomnia is the outcome.

The key ingredient in the Kales and Kales chronic insomnia hypothesis is predisposition, which is viewed in terms of extremes of a dimensional scale. People without chronic insomnia may have been exposed to the same provocation, but because of their lower predisposition (i.e., less extreme dimensional status as represented on MMPI assessments), they did not evolve the same persistent response.

A variety of subsequent insomnia research projects have used the MMPI and other personality instruments in the attempt to explain the vulnerability for chronic insomnia. For instance, Cynthia Dorsey and Richard Bootzin (1997) used the Eysenck Personality Inventory and found elevated neuroticism in a group of subjectively insomniac persons and increased introversion in an objectively insomniac group. Each group included insomnia complainers, but they differed in their perception of sleep during a daytime MSLT assessment. The investigators speculated that the subjectively insomniac persons experienced high levels of stress and anxiety, while the objectively insomniac persons were more ruminative and experienced increased cognitive arousal when attempting to sleep. The following case is consistent with this type of personality vulnerability.

Vicious Cycle Insomnia: Laura was a 47-year-old psychotherapist who was referred to the Sleep Disorders Center because of longstanding symptoms of insomnia. She also complained of excessive anxiety throughout her adult life, and she had been treated with intermittent outpatient psychotherapy and several trials with antidepressants. She remembered always having mild difficulty falling asleep, but she also had occasional episodes of marked sleep-onset difficulty lasting one to two weeks. She noted that these past episodes had been associated with stressful events. For four years now her sleep-onset insomnia had been persistent. She said that it began with work-related conflicts but that those problems were resolved years ago. Most recently, it had been taking her several hours to fall asleep, and some nights she was unable to sleep at all. She described herself as "hyperalert" throughout the daytime and increasingly anxious as bedtime approached due to her concern about whether she would get enough sleep. She said that she felt trapped in a "vicious cycle" of not being able to sleep because of her worry about not being able to sleep.

Another MMPI-based study of patients with chronic insomnia categorized the subjects into groups described as having psychologically based or medically based insomnia (Kalogjera-Sackellares and Cartwright, 1997). In both groups there was a high prevalence of psychopathology on MMPI scales, particularly indicating depression. The authors concluded that psychological factors additionally may be significant in patients with chronic insomnia that has other apparent causes.

The contributions of psychological factors to insomnia in relatively healthy elderly populations was emphasized by Beullens (1999) in a literature review. It was suggested that anxiety, neuroticism, and depression were greater among elderly insomnia sufferers. These psychological characteristics seemed to be more significant than were factors described as modes of living or health indicators.

Bliwise and colleagues (1995) used the NEO Personality Inventory to examine the outcomes of elderly insomnia patients treated with behavioral interventions (sleep-restriction therapy and relaxation training). While the NEO scores did not predict improvement in sleep onset, the subjects experiencing better outcomes in total sleep time tended to be "more traditional, conventional, and rigid."

Another dimensional psychological construct recently used in explanatory models of insomnia is *perfectionism.* Lundh and Broman (2000) argue that psychological processes increasing the vulnerability for insomnia can be classed as either sleep interfering or sleep interpreting. The sleep-interfering processes (e.g., stressful events, depression, and negative conditioning) result in cognitive or emotional arousal, which directly influences sleep. Sleep-interpreting processes relate to an individual's "personal standards, attitudes, beliefs, and fears" about sleep problems and potential consequences. The authors emphasize personal standards with regard to perfectionism. They suggest that a high degree of perfectionism may be an important vulnerability for insomnia, especially for the progression from transient to chronic insomnia.

The relationship of perfectionism and chronic insomnia also is examined by Vincent and Walker (2000), who consider the difference between adaptive and maladaptive perfectionism. They argue that maladaptive perfectionism may be associated with several disorders and symptoms, including insomnia. Maladaptive perfectionism is characterized by self-doubt, low self-esteem, excessive worry about performance, and an assumption that others have unreasonable expectations on the person. Vincent and Walker offer their findings in a study of subjects in chronic insomnia and control groups who completed multidimensional perfectionism scales. The characteristics of maladaptive perfectionism (concern over mistakes, frequent parental criticism, and doubts about action) were more likely in the group with chronic insomnia.

Dimensional psychological variables, such as those associated with internalization, neuroticism, introversion, and perfectionism constructs, have been the bases of insomnia investigations and theoretical models. These naturally lead to treatment implications. Individuals at the extremes of these dimensions are seen as having increased risk for insomnia due to these enduring vulnerabilities.

Summary

The dimensional perspective illuminates clinical situations by emphasizing enduring vulnerabilities to various problems that result from an individual being at an extreme end of a spectrum. The person's position along a dimensional scale signifies the potential for experiencing difficulty when faced with a provocation, which then influences the response, which may have clinical significance. These dimensions are features that exist to greater or lesser extents among individuals, and a person's position may be indicated by a direct measurement or indirectly through an instrument designed to represent a psychological construct.

Circadian rhythm phase predisposition is an enduring characteristic in adulthood, and it ranges from the early birds to the night owls, with most people in between and able to sleep normal hours. However, either of the extreme positions increases a person's vulnerability for the experience of insomnia. These advanced and delayed circadian phase tendencies commonly influence people with chronic insomnia and often are unrecognized as contributing to the person's vulnerability.

Personality features typically are defined along a spectrum and often are measured with an assortment of psychometric instruments to yield a score. This realm of variation in personality characteristics has been used widely to explain the predisposition for chronic insomnia. The psychological construct of internalization, whereby individuals do not directly express their feelings and emotional conflicts, can be construed with such instruments as the MMPI. It is argued that a greater degree of internalization explains why some people will recover fairly rapidly from a provocation-induced insomnia and others will develop a persistent pattern of chronic insomnia.

The dimensional perspective is especially valuable in highlighting one's risk for chronic insomnia. This viewpoint can help direct treatment guiding people toward positions of lower vulnerability. Depending on the identified predispositions, important components of an overall treatment approach may include psychotherapeutic strategies, particular behavioral changes, and perhaps manipulations of one's circadian rhythm.

5

Life as the Context of Sleep

Insomnia is an understandable response to life circumstances.

The Life-Story Perspective

Fundamentally, all clinical presentations involve story telling. There always is a narrative element to the description of symptoms. The story usually involves an account of when and how the particular complaint evolved and of what new life difficulties it may have created. Often the narrative provides the context of the problem, which may implicitly suggest an explanation, real or imagined. For instance: "These headaches began when I started my new job two years ago. They have been getting worse since then, and now I miss a few days of work each month because of them." The story might then continue with a discussion of the unreasonable supervisor, toxic environment, bad lighting, or stressful deadlines. In a clinical setting, the patient will be encouraged to detail the history further with facets of location, severity, specific time course, factors that aggravate or alleviate the symptom, and any other associated features. This type of clinical history is critical in generating a differential diagnosis, directing treatment strategies, and assessing outcomes. However, the clinical importance of the story is not confined to just this potential scientific value. Rather, the story is a greater embodiment of *this* problem in the context of *this* person's life.

This life-story method of understanding problems is both natural and familiar. We innately organize events temporally and attempt to explain how one thing causes another. We relate to others' circumstances, and we are sympathetic to their misfortunes. We can appreciate the uniqueness of a person and the characteristics he or she brings to a situation, and we can try to understand why the person responds as he or she does. This type of explanation is not necessarily synonymous with scientific models, and the question of accuracy may not even be relevant. McHugh and Slavney (1998) suggest that the logic of the life-story approach is that of the historical narrative, which presents a compelling account of settings, sequences, and outcomes. Essentially, it is persuasion—making the case for a particular interpretation. This historical method, ideally, involves a thorough and critical review of the facts, an appraisal of various interpretations, and a balanced presentation of conclusions, but there is some risk of bias throughout the process. Nevertheless, this historical approach potentially is quite powerful in offering explanation—identifying meaningful connections—regarding particular events and reactions and, in some cases, broad temporal trends or underlying forces.

In psychiatry, the life story plays a key role as it evolves in a psychotherapeutic relationship. The patient's personal history, constitutional characteristics, and various strengths and weaknesses provide the unique setting. The salient elements of the story sequence lead to the eventual outcomes: thoughts, moods, and behaviors. An effective story generates a sense of plausibility and inevitability, it offers explanation and meaning, and it guides the direction of the psychotherapy and the overall treatment approach. The story flows from the patient, perhaps with interpretation from the therapist. Dominant patterns and themes may emerge in the story but should not be imposed on it. That is, the patient's setting can lead to the symptom outcome, but the opposite should not be assumed: the presence of particular symptoms does not automatically presuppose a setting and sequence of events. Adherents of particular schools of thought in psychiatry find value in the associated explanatory models but risk bias if they work backward by assuming that a symptom always has the same precipitants. We appreciate that childhood sexual abuse can lead to adult psychopathology; however, the presence of adult psychopathology in a particular individual does not mean that he or she experienced childhood sexual abuse.

There is great potential therapeutic value inherent in the life-story method. First, it is satisfying in that it emphasizes the uniqueness of the individual. Second, the sense of explanation is reassuring. Third, the story may identify things that can be changed and, therefore, can provide hope for the future. There may be habitual responses to situations that can be altered. And, since the story is not over, it can be rescripted for the future as part of the therapeutic process.

There are as many stories of insomnia as there are people suffering from insomnia. In fact, there are many more: each person's unique setting and symptoms can be viewed and interpreted, and the case formulated, in very different ways and, consequently, with an assortment of stories. These individual stories can highlight one's risk factors, personality vulnerabilities, and problematic habits, as well as the onset of related disorders and subsequent reactions. And while these stories provide meaning for individuals and therapists and can help guide treatment, just as importantly, more general themes can emerge from the collective body of cases. Indeed, this life-story-narrative approach is the foundation of the leading contemporary explanatory models of insomnia and is the underpinning of the primary treatment modalities currently employed.

The Single Sleep Story

In terms of life experience, insomnia is universal. Therefore, to some degree at least, everyone can relate to the frustration of sleeplessness. Insomnia is a familiar story element and an understandable outcome in various narratives of misfortune, illness, distress, and excitement, as well as in the narrative context of medical and psychiatric disorders. Consider the following:

- "Yesterday my boss told me my performance was inadequate and I was being demoted. I couldn't sleep at all last night."
- "I've been so depressed the last few weeks. I just don't want to be alive anymore. I can hardly eat anything and I seem to wake up every hour during the night."
- "Whenever I'm on call, I keep waiting for the beeper to go off. Even on a quiet night I can't relax and sleep soundly."
- "I've been having the worst time getting to sleep ever since this back pain started."
- "I shouldn't have had that coffee after dinner, because I couldn't fall asleep until almost dawn."

These minicases have familiar situations and outcomes ranging from acute to chronic. We readily accept insomnia resulting from a great variety of disturbances. The above stories easily could be expanded into detailed narratives, but even in this brief form there is a sense of plausibility, perhaps inevitability. Each of these individual insomnia stories makes sense, not so much with testable scientific logic, but through narrative logic explanation. When bad things happen, it is not surprising to hear that insomnia is one of the results.

> *The Terrorized Wife:* Delores was a 50-year-old professional woman who had always slept well until about three years before her Sleep Center evaluation. She began to experience severe difficulty falling and remaining asleep. Ultimately, she felt so impaired during the daytime that she obtained disability for these symptoms. She associated the onset of the sleep difficulty with persistent terrorizing behaviors from her now ex-husband. She elaborated a wide variety of vicious behaviors and threats beginning immediately after their marriage and continuing after their divorce. Her husband had developed several intricate schemes to maintain her in a constant state of fear. These involved not just a directly aggressive stance but also stalking behavior and the creation of situations purposely to frighten her. Ultimately, she was forced to take legal action and even to move to a secret location. Recently, she had been going to bed around 11:00 P.M., but usually it had taken her several hours to fall asleep. At that point her sleep would be very light and she experienced frequent awakenings. She estimated getting less than four hours of sleep per night. She described tossing and turning, as well as talking very actively in her sleep. Her sleep also was punctuated with very distressing nightmare awakenings. She had tried a variety of over-the-counter and prescription hypnotics, all with limited benefit. She felt that she now was able to put the horrifying episode with the ex-husband behind her, but she remained distressed about her impairment due to the nighttime and daytime effects of her insomnia.

In a very general sense, and recognizing that there should be considerable individual variation in vulnerability to insomnia, we would expect a positive correlation between the intensity of distress and the likelihood and severity of a sleep disturbance outcome. Indeed, the individual life stories that might be described with the contemporary label of posttraumatic stress disorder are required to demonstrate increased arousal, very commonly manifest by insomnia symptoms.

With this life-story approach to insomnia, it is possible to elaborate the context of the person's symptoms. This is a huge domain and may include such features as family and personal history, personality features, habitual routines, schedules, attitudes, expectations, medical and psychiatric history, medications, a thorough description of the sleep complaint (onset, duration, timing, etc.), treatment attempts (successes and failures), and the ramifications of the sleep difficulty. The insomnia story from the patient, and perhaps expanded and further interpreted in a psychotherapeutic setting, attempts to explain why *this* person has *this* experience of insomnia at *this* time. The story implicitly may incorporate one or more hypotheses, some of which may imply specific therapeutic avenues. For instance, the story might propose that to improve sleep one might need to deal more effectively with job stressors, treat an underlying mood disorder, optimize treatment of medical disorders and improve pain management, and/or stop evening consumption of caffeine. The story explanation may suggest an easy habit change (caffeine), a more challenging solution (treatment of medical and psychiatric disorders), a long-term psychotherapy plan (better coping with workplace conflicts), or, perhaps, that the identified underlying problem cannot be changed and the insomnia must be addressed in another manner (e.g., hypnotics). In *No More Sleepless Nights,* sleep disorders specialist Peter Hauri emphasizes the importance of hypothesis building and experimentation with different treatment strategies in the process of treating insomnia patients (Hauri, Linde, and Westbrook, 1996). The patient and clinician longitudinally monitor the effectiveness of each strategy with a sleep diary. There is no problem with story changes, just as scientific explanation may meander with new evidence.

Various instruments have been developed in the attempt to quantify the number and severity of defined stressful life events experienced by a person during a period of time. An obvious hypothesis is that a score representing greater distress should predict greater sleep disturbance. Several studies have compared populations of normal and disturbed sleepers using such scales. One example was that of Anthony Kales and colleagues (Healey et al., 1981), who rated life-stress events with the Schedule of Recent Experience in controls and in poor sleepers during the index year of insomnia onset, as well as in each of the two years before and after the onset. Consistent with the hypothesis, the poor sleepers were much more likely to have a higher stress score, particularly with undesirable events, such as those related to losses or ill health. The researchers found that 75 percent of the poor sleepers associated the onset of their disturbance with a stressful life event. Of course, this reflects the person's own narrative explanation.

Although a life story easily can be reduced to a bare outline that can represent a compelling case of why someone might sleep poorly, a major strength of this approach is that it can emphasize the role of the individual. It is natural to sympathize with the concerns of the woman in the following case.

> *The Russian Worrier:* Sasha, a 48-year-old woman, presented to the Sleep Center because of persistent nighttime awakenings. She had been born and raised in Russia, where she had been educated through an advanced degree in the clinical sciences. She was married and had two children doing well in college. She and her immediate family had immigrated to the United States four years previously. She and her husband had secured job positions appropriate to their high level of training. She reported that she had had difficulty with her sleep during stressful times, mostly job related, beginning soon after she had moved from Russia. At the time of the evaluation, her sleep had been very disturbed persistently for six months, and she attributed this to her worries concerning her father's health, as he was diagnosed with cancer at that time. Since he had remained in Russia, she would telephone him at what for her was the middle of the night. Most nights she was rather sleepy at her 11:00 P.M. bedtime, and she would fall asleep quickly. However, she usually would awaken within two hours, at which time she felt rather anxious and would ruminate about assorted problems. If she was able to get any more sleep, it was repeatedly disrupted. She was out of bed for the day between 6:00 and 7:00 A.M. Throughout the daytime she felt fatigued and had difficulty concentrating. She was frustrated about her distressing nighttime experiences and her impaired functioning during the daytime.

Narrative explanation is abundant in Sasha's insomnia history. Distress about her father's illness, her nighttime telephone calls, and worry about her daytime performance all can be viewed as contributing to her disturbed sleep.

The following patient presented not because of current insomnia but rather because of fear of a recurrence of past insomnia. Life choices often affect insomnia; here, insomnia influenced life choices.

> *The Fear of Not Sleeping:* Paula was a 30-year-old, married woman who came to the Sleep Disorders Center because of her worry about a return of insomnia, which in the past had been quite distressing for her. Her difficulty with insomnia had begun four years previously, after the birth of her only child, a daughter. At that time she had felt rather depressed and had experienced frequent tearful episodes. The depression disappeared

within a few weeks, and soon after that the baby was sleeping well at nighttime. However, distressing sleeplessness continued. Paula's obstetrician prescribed pentobarbital and then flurazepam, which usually was helpful and which she continued to take about once a month. Most nights she was able to fall asleep quickly at her 11:00 P.M. bedtime and then sleep soundly until 7:00 A.M. She felt alert and energetic during the daytime. The immediate concern prompting the evaluation was her desire to become pregnant again, and her feeling "petrified" of the return of the insomnia, especially as she assumed that she would not be able to take hypnotics. One year before the evaluation, she had become pregnant, but she had elected to have an abortion rather than risk suffering the distressing insomnia again.

Sleep Hygiene

Insomnia sufferers, their confidants, and their health care providers may identify particular behaviors they think might be a cause of the sleeplessness; thus, changing the behavior might result in a cure. Sleep hygiene is a general description often used to describe a body of advice related to presumably sleep-friendly behaviors. Lists of sleep hygiene recommendations typically include such items as limiting caffeine and alcohol, avoiding excessive evening exercise, and developing relaxing bedtime routines. There is an implied narrative logic: "You have insomnia because of something you are doing." Essentially, sleep hygiene involves insomnia short-story-therapeutic paradigms: Stop doing x or start doing y, and subsequently you will sleep better. Both x and y usually are specific behaviors that presumably can influence the undesired outcome—insomnia. Of course, since there are many insomnia stories, what is relevant for one person may be less meaningful for another. Furthermore, with sleep hygiene advice being quite generalized, what might be therapeutic in one clinical situation could have the opposite effect for another person. The potential therapeutic value of sleep hygiene is discussed further in chapter 7.

The Bedtime Story

Although insomnia is a common complaint, more people report generally sleeping well than those who complain about their sleep. Good and poor sleepers may follow identical routines in preparation for sleep, yet the outcomes differ. Evening and bedtime routines seem to reinforce sleep onset for good sleepers.

> *The Bedtime Reader:* A 48-year-old sleep specialist typically falls asleep at his usual bedtime without difficulty. After his habitual bedtime preparations, but before turning out the light, he enjoys reading briefly—often very briefly, perhaps only a paragraph. Then, on turning out the light, sleep ensues rapidly. He considers the reading a very comfortable activity, and he senses that skipping that step would leave a gap and perhaps lengthen his sleep latency.

Consistent with behaviorist conditioning theory, just about any bedtime ritual could reinforce sleep onset in the good sleeper. Seemingly trivial sleep-enhancing bedtime routines can be taken for granted with regard to their power in supporting a satisfying sleep onset experience.

> *Praying for Sleep:* A five-year-old boy generally sleeps very well. With support from his parents, he follows a regular evening and bedtime routine. The evening evolves with eating a snack, brushing his teeth, getting washed up and into pajamas, briefly reading in the bedroom with a parent, turning lights out (nightlight on), saying prayers, sharing a goodnight kiss, parent leaving, and sleep happening. The boy always is faithful about completing his prayers and, surely not from disrespect or boredom, invariably yawns wonderfully in the middle of the prayers.

Like the other elements in the progression of the evening routine, the prayers can be interpreted as regularly being associated with sleep onset and therefore can be seen as a reinforcing cue.

The woman described below has felt that she has a dependency on a particular bedtime sleep-onset cue, without which she cannot easily fall asleep.

> *TV Addiction:* This 36-year-old, married, professional woman reported that throughout her adult life she often found it difficult to fall asleep. Once asleep, usually she could remain asleep until her normal morning wakeup time. Most days she functioned fine, but after an especially bad night, she felt very fatigued and had difficulty concentrating. Although she felt that she had a good relationship with her husband, she had given up trying to fall asleep in bed with him. She had evolved a routine of going to the family room, watching television, and then falling asleep without

much difficulty. She felt completely dependent on falling asleep while the 11:30 P.M. *M*A*S*H* reruns were playing. She noticed sleepiness with the familiar theme music, and often she was asleep within a few minutes. Since the reruns were broadcast nightly, this routine seemed to work well for her. On the occasions when the broadcast was preempted, she had much more difficulty falling asleep. The pattern continued for many years, but eventually the *M*A*S*H* rerun broadcasts were discontinued. She then experienced nightly difficulty with sleep onset. Only after many months was she able to fall asleep comfortably with reruns of another nightly situation comedy.

If the bedtime and the bedroom (more specifically, the bed) are the immediate time and place for sleep, then they are likewise for insomnia. Accordingly, they can play leading roles in insomnia narratives. It is easy to posit that the sleep environment that works positively for the good sleeper can work negatively for the insomniac person. This context of sleeplessness can be viewed as having developed a detrimental role— promoting persistent insomnia. In the next insomnia story, Jean first reacts to distressing news with sleeplessness and then seems to respond to her bedroom with sleeplessness.

The Vacation Sleeper: Jean, a 68-year-old woman, presented to the Sleep Disorders Center because of her severe difficulty falling asleep during the previous three years. The symptoms began at the time of her retirement and also when she was diagnosed with metastases from previous breast cancer. She was regarded as doing well medically at the time of her sleep evaluation. During the past few years, she found that, in spite of going to bed much earlier, she was unable to fall asleep until around 3:00 A.M., and she would awaken spontaneously between 6:00 and 7:00 A.M. She avoided napping during the daytime, although she did feel rather sleepy. Recently, she had been involved in two automobile accidents resulting from her drowsy driving. She had evolved an evening routine of retiring to her bedroom about 8:00 P.M. Sitting in the bed with the television turned on, she would pay bills, attend to correspondence, read, and talk on the phone. Eventually, she would just watch television and, after several frustrating hours, finally fall asleep. Over the previous two months, she had been away with friends on three vacation trips averaging one week each. She discovered that she was able to sleep quite well during all of these trips. She was rather surprised that she slept a solid eight hours on a few nights. On returning home each time, her sleep immediately deteriorated.

The elaboration of a narrative-logic explanation in Jean's case could include a psychological process whereby she has come to associate her own bedroom with the inability to sleep. She sleeps better away from home because she is not exposed to the familiar home cues for sleeplessness. The exact opposite situation exists in the following story of a young man who believes that he can sleep only in the ideal environment that he can create in his own bedroom.

> **The Perfect Sleeper:** Tim was a 30-year-old, single man who came to the Sleep Disorders Center because of his concern about not being able to sleep well while traveling. He was successful and happy in his occupation, and he was active socially and athletically. A few months previously he had accepted a job that required a few days of traveling away from home each week. He had been sleeping very poorly those nights, and he felt that his daytime performance was suffering. In fact, he had fallen asleep during business meetings. He had known for several years that sleep away from his own bedroom always was a great problem. This included occasional work-related travel as well as visits to his parent's home. In his own bedroom in his apartment, he was confident that he would sleep fine, as long as he created what he termed the right "zone." This included a rather cool temperature and the use of a comforter on the bed, complete darkness and the use of eyeshades, and a bedside fan for white noise, as well as careful attention to his scheduled hours for sleep. With these items in place, he slept well from his midnight bedtime until a spontaneous awakening about 8:00 A.M. and he felt fully alert and productive during the following day. Away from his bedroom, he estimated that he had been able to get only four to five hours of very light sleep and then had felt terrible the next day. He also had found that he had been unable to sleep with anyone else in bed with him. Previously, he had lived with a girlfriend for several months. He arranged for them to sleep in adjacent, separate beds, which allowed him a sufficient amount of sleep.

What is the explanation for this situation where a young man is suffering and seeking help because he can sleep well only in his own bedroom—ideally while alone? Clearly, his bedroom is a key element in the narrative logic, as are the assorted preparations he makes to create his sleep "zone." No doubt, conditioning must play some role. One might suggest further that he sleeps well, in part, because he minimizes environmental disturbances. Perhaps, having the sense that he has prepared the correct milieu, he is not anxious about a bad sleep outcome and actually has a sense of confidence about his ability to sleep that night or any night, under the right circumstances.

This question of confidence, its presence or absence and its relation to good sleep or insomnia, can be viewed as a major underlying theme in the greater realm of insomnia explanation. A lack of confidence about the ability to sleep, a sense of helplessness about the problem, and even a feeling of victimization because of the insomnia frequently can be heard in the stories of chronic insomnia sufferers. It is a compelling story, it is plausible, and it is very useful because it does provide explanation and can help direct treatment—psychotherapeutic and behavioral. However, it is the narrative logic of the life-story approach that underlies the explanation, not an understanding derived from a precise diagnostic test or criterion. In fact, this appreciation of insomnia does not depend on diagnosis at all. It may be valuable with patients given an assortment of sleep-related diagnoses, and treatment emanating from this formulation can blend well with other strategies directed at solving the sleep disturbance. This assumes, of course, that the individual patient has been evaluated thoroughly with regard to potential factors influencing the insomnia complaint and that premature conclusions have not caused important contributing elements to be neglected.

Theory and Therapy

The life-story approach offers explanation not just for individuals but also for groups of people who can be viewed as sharing rather general story elements or processes related to their complaints of insomnia. Trends may be identified, broad themes can be described, and, sometimes, theoretical orientations will emerge. Theories of insomnia causation, as well as types of insomnia and even specific diagnostic categories, can be posited from this more global consideration of collective bodies of insomnia narratives. Therapeutic strategies addressing the identified causes then can be proposed. The potential value is great: explanation and treatment for large groups of insomnia sufferers.

Some caution is necessary in this process of forming an insomnia theory and in the application of the implicit treatment strategies. There is danger of excessively broad attribution—that is, assuming that the presence of insomnia symptoms presupposes a particular developmental narrative, which, as suggested above, is working backward. A disproportionate attachment to a theoretical orientation can restrict the breadth of potential contributing factors considered in a particular case. Some practitioners will view the outcome—insomnia, presume the history of a depressive disorder, and consequently always prescribe an antidepressant medication. Others almost always will turn to particular psychotherapeutic and/or behavioral strategies. With insomnia complaints, only rarely is there a particular test or a decisively defined diagnosis to guide the practitioner with great precision toward an explanation and a detailed treatment plan. (An exceptional example would be a low serum ferritin level increasing the risk for restless legs syndrome, which may promote sleep-onset difficulty and which may be treated with iron supplementation.) But, in spite of the intrinsic diagnostic weaknesses associated with insomnia, treatment approaches still can be evaluated carefully with scientific methods analyzing outcome measures.

The following very brief case examples easily lead to formulations that represent major themes in the explanation and treatment of insomnia:

- "I almost never sleep. I'm not sleepy at 8:00 P.M., but I get in bed by then because I know it will take me hours to fall asleep. I get out of bed about 8:00 A.M., but I know that I've only had a few hours of sleep and I feel terrible."
- "I'm sleepy in the evening, but when my head hits the pillow my mind is racing and I'm wide awake. This has been going on for months now for no reason."
- "I know that I'll feel awful if I don't get enough sleep tonight. I just don't know what I'm going to do. I can't go on like this."

Three contemporary dominant themes in the theory and therapy of chronic insomnia symptoms revolve around what generally are described as sleep restriction, stimulus control, and cognitive-behavioral therapeutic approaches. Each of these explanatory models fundamentally has a narrative basis. The insomnia sufferer thought to benefit from an approach is presumed to have evolved the insomnia outcome as a result of the setting and sequence, (i.e., the individual circumstances and events that have evolved over time). The formulating theme for one person's chronic insomnia interpretation represents a general template of explanation centered on the theoretical orientation. Treatment is directed at correcting the underlying problem, which is shared with many other insomnia patients. The narrative-logic significance in this process of insomnia explanation is all the more evident considering the rather broad applicability of the approaches. These models do make sense, and the associated treatments are efficacious. However, they are more driven by story than by diagnosis. With none of these approaches is there a precise diagnostic test or criterion suggesting exactly what groups of individuals would or would not benefit from the particular treatment strategy. Furthermore, these approaches are not at all mutually exclusive and, in clinical practice settings, commonly are combined (Stepanski, 2000).

Sleep Restriction

Restriction of the time in bed, thereby limiting the time available for sleep, is the essence of the sleep restriction therapeutic approach, which has been advanced by Arthur Spielman (Spielman, Saskin, and Thorpy, 1987). The underlying argument is that many people with chronic insomnia, in the evolution of their sleep disturbance, have come to spend excessive time in bed most nights and that this behavior then has had a detrimental effect on their ability to experience sufficient and refreshing sleep. In extreme cases, they may be in bed with hopes of sleeping, as opposed to using the bed for various other activities, for extraordinary and unrealistic periods— 12 hours or more nightly. Alternatively, they may be in bed a normal amount of time, but if they are sleeping much less than that, they still end up with considerable wakeful time in bed. Excessive time in bed usually results from the belief that it is the only way to get whatever amount of sleep might be afforded them that night. Many insomniac persons believe that they are supposed to be in bed throughout the normal nighttime sleep hours. They fear missing any opportunity during which sleep might occur. They may think that they must stay in bed at least to rest their bodies, or they may remain there to avoid bothering others in the house, from embarrassment about the insomnia, or because they cannot think of anything else to do at that hour.

The sleep restriction premise is that excessive wakeful time in bed during attempts to sleep has the effect of perpetuating the symptoms of insomnia. Those spending extraordinary amounts of time in bed set themselves up for failure. Inevitably, they will be awake for portions of the night, since homeostatically they will not be able to sleep for such extended periods. The sleep restriction plan actually takes advantage of the homeostatic sleep drive by temporarily inducing mild sleep deprivation.

Although sleep restriction therapy has been used with variations, the basic strategy is to limit the time in bed to the amount of time the individual estimates he or she is sleeping according to a nightly sleep log. Time in bed never is curtailed to less than four and one-half hours. According to circadian principles, a normal morning arising time is kept stable throughout the treatment, and the hours in bed are determined by the scheduled bedtime. As the sleep log demonstrates improvement in sleep during the allotted time in bed, then the bedtime gradually may be advanced earlier. The initial guidelines suggested that, when one sleeps at least 90 percent of the scheduled time for five nights, then the bedtime is to be advanced 15 minutes earlier. However, if sleep time has dropped below 85 percent, then the bedtime would be delayed. Napping is not permitted. The goal, of course, is to minimize wakeful time in bed. This is accomplished with the curtailed sleep time allotment and is enhanced with the extra sleepiness resulting from the restriction. During the therapeutic process, the insomnia-perpetuating factors associated with wakeful time in bed will be diminished, so an improved sleep experience eventually can be achieved.

While the focus of sleep restriction is the therapeutic strategy, it presupposes the historical narrative of the vulnerable individual sleeping poorly, spending too much wakeful time in bed, and thereby sustaining the insomnia. This is not dependent on an exacting diagnostic process, although many insomnia patients treated with this approach probably are labeled with the diagnosis of psychophysiological insomnia or primary insomnia. It is the temporal sequence that presumably has contributed to the chronic insomnia outcome that is being reversed with the restricted time in bed. Therefore, sleep restriction may be effective with a variety of patients and in combination with other treatment approaches.

Stimulus Control

The mental association between going to bed and not sleeping is at the core of the stimulus control approach, which has been associated primarily with the work of Richard Bootzin and colleagues (Bootzin and Nicassio, 1978). For whatever reason, perhaps a very understandable life event, the vulnerable person experiences symptoms of insomnia. With time, and possibly rather quickly, going to bed—that is, the bedtime hour, the intention to attempt sleeping, the bedroom and bed, and all of the bedtime routines that should be positive cues for sleep—becomes associated with sleeplessness. There may be a dread of bedtime approaching, along with increasing performance anxiety as the anticipated hour nears. Once in bed, there might be a feeling of having a racing mind, frustration, and even agitation about the sleeplessness. One can posit both cognitive and physiological aspects to this hyperaroused experience, which is reinforced by the nightly bedtime stimuli. It seems logical that, as the insomniac person spends more time awake in this dysphoric and aroused state, the association between preparing for and being in bed, on the one hand, and this sleepless mental state, on the other, is further strengthened. The maintained association of bed with an inability to sleep predicts a return of this conditioned response on subsequent nights. This pattern is most apparent in the insomnia sufferers who may feel sleepy and nod off downstairs in the evening while watching television but find that their eyes are wide open and their minds are racing by the time they get in bed and their heads hit the pillow. This conditioned hyperaroused state can occur, as well, with nighttime awakenings. While brief awakenings during the night are normal, a conditioned hyperarousal easily can undermine a rapid return to sleep. The result then may be extended and frustrating wakeful episodes during the night.

Once again, there is a basic narrative logic in the sequence of events and the insomnia outcome. And again, there is an attempt to reverse the process—with this approach, by controlling or limiting the conditioned hyperarousing stimuli. This generalized conditioning process contributing to persistent insomnia makes a compelling explanation, which can be conceived in the cases of many individuals with insomnia symptoms. The presumption of the process, rather than a specific diagnosis, suggests the therapy, although, as with the sleep restriction approach, many patients will have been labeled with diagnoses of psychophysiological or primary insomnia.

Deconditioning is the essential desired action of stimulus-control therapy. The goal must be the elimination of the ongoing reinforcement between the constellation of elements constituting the sleep environment and the hyperarousal that now inhibits a satisfying sleep experience. Generally, this means minimizing wakeful time in bed. Typical instructions include not going to bed until one is sleepy and feeling able to fall asleep. If one experiences the hyperaroused and frustrated state or simply remains awake for more than about 10 minutes, one is to leave the bed and attempt sleep again later. Similarly, this can apply to nighttime awakenings. As with the sleep restriction approach, the scheduled morning wakeup time remains constant, and napping is avoided.

Although the stimulus control and sleep restriction approaches have different theoretical bases, in practice there is some overlap. With stimulus control there may be temporary sleep deprivation that subsequently may have a beneficial effect in enhancing sleep onset. Intrinsic to the sleep restriction plan is avoidance of excessive wakeful time in bed, and therefore it incorporates some degree of stimulus control. And while these two approaches are based on generalized temporal processes, for the individual there is the story-based explanation that now can change with renewed hope of improved sleep. The story can be redirected, with the insomnia sufferer shifting from the role of victim to the agent of change.

Cognitive-Behavioral Therapy

Among the major current psychotherapeutic approaches is cognitive-behavioral therapy, which evolved from the work of Aaron Beck and Albert Ellis. The organizing principle is that one's feelings and behaviors are derived from the mental structures of one's experiences. Faulty cognitions, beliefs, and assumptions are seen as causing certain types of psychopathology. Various cognitive errors can be described as overgeneralization, dichotomous thinking, catastrophizing, maximizing and minimizing, selective abstraction, and personalization. Cognitive-behavioral therapy, then, involves an interactive psychotherapy directed at identifying and correcting the cognitive distortions and dysfunctional beliefs and at promoting the modification of maladaptive behaviors. This approach has been used widely in the treatment of symptoms, including depression, anxiety, phobias, obsessions, and compulsions.

Strategies derived from the cognitive-behavioral orientation have been adapted to the problem of insomnia. A major proponent in the sleep arena has been Charles Morin (1993). Although the conceptual basis regarding insomnia clearly is distinct, the application is rather broad and freely takes advantage of sleep hygiene, sleep restriction, and stimulus control recom-

mendations. The narrative logic of the cognitive-behavioral approach con-
centrates on the process of insomnia development and maintenance due
to cognitive distortions—dysfunctional beliefs and attitudes regarding
sleep need and the consequences of insufficient sleep. It is argued that
both unrealistic expectations and irrational fears function to promote
increased tension and anxiety and, therefore, sleeplessness. These factors
may heighten one's vulnerability to insomnia and certainly exacerbate the
symptoms once an episode has begun. Individuals with chronic insomnia
tend to ruminate, with decidedly negative content, throughout the daytime
and increasingly as bedtime approaches. There seems to be a self-fulfill-
ing prophecy in the anticipation of sleepless misery. If this nightly mental
scenario can be rescripted, then the future story can be changed and there
can be a new outcome—satisfying sleep. The goal of the treatment, then,
is to deflate the arousing mental routine through the correction and redi-
rection of the cognitive distortions.

Ideally, the cognitive-behavioral approach to chronic insomnia is
through a series of therapy sessions that focus on sleep education, healthy
sleep practices, corrections of maladaptive cognitions, and a review of the
progress thus far achieved. Maladaptive behaviors, such as excessive time
in bed, irregular schedules, and napping, can be addressed, and sleep-
friendly behaviors can be encouraged. The goal is for this short-term therapy to have long-term efficacy, since the corrected cognitions and
behaviors will leave the individual less vulnerable to future insomnia.

Psychotherapy

While cognitive-behavioral therapy is a specific type of psychotherapy,
other psychotherapeutic strategies also may play valuable roles in the
treatment of insomnia symptoms. Issues related to personality vulnerabilities, life stressors, and factors reinforcing chronic insomnia, as well as the
consequences of the sleep disturbance, all can be addressed, and perhaps
resolved, through psychotherapeutic approaches. Narrative logic forms
the basis of explanation in psychotherapy. In some cases a patient's life
story that promotes persistent distress, anxiety, helplessness, and insomnia can be rescripted so that he or she can take an active role in recovery.
It is a powerful therapeutic transition for the patient to emerge from victimhood to agent of change.

Pharmacotherapy

Although hypnotics and other medications used to help with sleep act primarily on neurotransmitter receptor sites and not plot lines, these treatment approaches, nevertheless, often become prominent elements in a patient's insomnia story. Certainly, any past therapeutic successes and failures are important in the clinical history. Medications also may take on symbolic roles with particular expectations, beliefs, attitudes, and fears. These may be influenced by past experience or may be derived from family, friends, and media reports. Some patients will present with the weighty history of having tried all imaginable somnogenic agents: herbals, over-the-counter antihistamines, multiple hypnotics, and most available antidepressants. They then may implicitly challenge the health care provider now to prescribe just the right medication to cure instantly their chronic sleep disturbance. In other cases, however, the institution of hypnotic therapy will provide psychological relief along with the active sedative effect.

The Three Ps

The consideration of predisposing, precipitating, and perpetuating factors related to insomnia has become universal in the field of sleep medicine, thanks to the writings of Arthur Spielman (Spielman, Saskin, and Thorpy, 1987). This is not a representation of a particular theoretical orientation; rather, it is a global model of compelling narrative logic regarding the evolution of insomnia symptoms. Individual stories explaining insomnia easily can be presented with this model, which may help guide the clinician in identifying relevant factors in a particular case. With chronic insomnia, this inherently temporal framework parallels the McHugh and Slavney life-story triad as predisposing factors represent the setting, precipitants relate to the sequence, and perpetuation is the outcome.

Everyone can be seen as having some degree of predisposition to insomnia, perhaps due to personality vulnerabilities, circadian rhythm tendency, and lifestyle. Generally, this may be thought of as one's intrinsic arousability. One or more immediate factors may be identified as contributing directly to the onset of the insomnia episode. Typically, these might include situational crises, medical and psychiatric illnesses, effects of medications and other substances, and schedule changes. The common feature is that there is a new or increased stress. Ideally, the insomnia will end with the resolution of the acute precipitant. The key idea in this model, however, is that in some situations new perpetuating factors will sustain the sleep disturbance, thereby creating a chronic insomnia. In other words, whatever started the insomnia may no longer be relevant to its continuation. Perpetuating culprits may be quite varied. For example, poor nighttime sleep sometimes can lead to a routine of daily napping, which then contributes to further poor nighttime sleep. Or poor sleep might lead one to use alcohol at bedtime, which then contributes to further sleep disruption later during the night. The conditioned hyperarousal of the stimulus control approach provides another example of a newly emerged sustaining factor. The evolution of cognitive distortions also may perpetuate insomnia. Overall, this framework highlights potential insomnia influences at different times and at different parts of the narrative.

Cultural Considerations

Just as one's life circumstances, and thereby one's life story, are the context of sleep, one's culture is an important context of one's life. Thus, culture may have a great influence on many aspects of sleep, including locations, family sleeping arrangements, bedtime routines, schedules, expectations, and even the definition of what is normal sleep. Cultural factors, therefore, can significantly affect the experience of sleep, whether it is considered abnormal, and how one might explain a disruption of sleep. Further, culture will have an effect on whether one complains of a sleep problem and on what one might do to solve it.

In the following case, it is evident that a wide assortment of stories can be constructed to explain the patient's initial and persistent difficulty with sleep; however, her cultural beliefs clearly influence her own explanation and the strategies she pursues to improve her sleep.

> *Evil Eye Insomnia:* Nina was a 28-year-old woman who was born and raised in Bulgaria and, at the time of her evaluation in the Sleep Center, had been in the United States for three years. She was actively working on a business degree in college and also had full-time employment. She had been in a relationship with a boyfriend for 18 months, and she hoped to marry him eventually. Her psychiatric history included a diagnosis of panic disorder beginning at age 19; however, she had been treated with

medications only during the past 18 months. She had tried a variety of antidepressants and now for about one year had been on doxepin, 25 mg three times a day, with good results.

She reported that throughout her life she never had any difficulty with her sleep, but she did tend to be a night person. However, beginning six months previously, she had started to have severe and persistent problems falling asleep. She found that she would be sleepy in the evening, and sometimes she would nod off while watching television, but as bedtime approached she would become increasingly anxious. She described feeling afraid of going to bed because of the distress she anticipated. Once she got in bed around 11:00 P.M. to midnight, it would take her two to three hours to fall asleep.

The onset of the sleep difficulty corresponded with several events. At that time she had begun working in a bakery, which required her to be there at 4:00 A.M. She was very worried about how she would get enough sleep. Within a few months she was able to return to a position with a normal work schedule. Also, at the time of the onset of insomnia, there was a change in her ongoing treatment of allergies, and she was given a steroid injection. Finally, at the same time she had had temporary conflicts with her boyfriend and with another female friend. Recently, she had avoided all caffeine and alcohol, and she had found some relief with occasional use of prescribed hypnotics.

In spite of her presentation of the above temporal associations, however, she believed that the actual underlying cause of her insomnia was a witchcraft spell that had been placed on her several months previously by an older woman whom she knew to be very spiritual and to have the ability to cast spells. She felt that this was an exacerbation of an evil eye curse placed on her as a young child. About three weeks before the Sleep Center evaluation, Nina spoke with the spiritual woman and asked her to pray for her sleep to improve and to remove the curse. The patient then followed the traditional custom of wearing a shirt for several days, giving it to someone to pray over, and then having it returned so she again could sleep in it. She had the spiritual woman pray over a shirt, and she also sent several back to Bulgaria to be prayed over by other spiritually powerful women there. She still awaited their return but already had experienced some improvement in her sleep after wearing the locally prayed-over shirt. Nina was hopeful that the curse would be completely removed and that she soon would sleep normally again.

In Nina's case it is easy to identify such factors as her panic disorder, mild tendency to phase delay, acute change in work schedule, steroid use, and relationship conflicts as potentially contributing to the onset of the insomnia episode. A conditioned hyperarousal probably contributed to the perpetuation of the symptoms. Her explanation of the cause of her distressing insomnia episode as resulting from spells being placed on her, as well as her therapeutic strategy of having her shirts prayed over, clearly reveals her cultural traditions. We can interpret further that her individual vulnerabilities and the external precipitants helped initiate the insomnia, which subsequently was reinforced psychologically. Initially, she felt rather helpless—a victim of the spell. However, once she felt that she was directly addressing the root of the problem, she began to experience improvement. Of course, she also made positive changes in sleep hygiene and schedule.

The literature on culture and sleep is rather sparse. Some ethnographic reports deal with sleeping behaviors, and a few studies examine the frequency of insomnia complaints among different ethnic groups. An exception is the broad cross-cultural view on sleep offered by Worthman and Melby (2002). They discuss the ecology of sleep, including the physical environment (bedding, housing structure, presence of fire), social aspects (who sleeps where and with whom, child care responsibilities), and the biotic context (predators, parasites, and pests). Further, they argue that a society's technology and subsistence patterns, as well as social patterns, ritual practices, and beliefs about sleep (and what we call dreams), influence the individual sleep experience—positively or negatively. For instance, in some cultures there is a fear of sleep due to the perceived risk of control by outside forces, such as spirits.

Worthman and Melby point out that the sleep conditions typical in contemporary Western industrial societies are vastly different from how people currently sleep in other parts of the world and, presumably, how they have slept through history. The typical Western sleep practice and view of an ideal sleep environment is one that is highly secure and climate controlled with minimal external sensory stimulation and that emphasizes the solitary, not social, sleep experience. We promote rigid boundaries in terms of the appropriate time, place, and circumstances for sleep, whereas the boundaries for all of these domains in most other cultures are much more diffuse. These sleep norms define abnormality within a culture. Whether the inability to achieve satisfying sleep is actually a common experience or a major concern in other societies simply is not known. From this anthropological vantage, however, one can question to what degree the high rate of insomnia in our society is culturally influenced. Is insomnia part of the story of industrial Western society?

With this far-reaching cross-cultural view of sleep, Worthman and Melby contribute to a recent question debated in the field of sleep research: What is normal sleep, or is there a single normality of sleep? More specifically, did humans evolve with a single, consolidated nighttime sleep episode of about eight hours—our sleep ideal—or is this model pattern of the solid, uninterrupted nightly sleep an artificial product of our culture—one that might have inherent vulnerabilities and therefore be difficult to maintain. From this point of view, what we would consider to be insomnia—particularly extended wakeful periods during the night—might represent the norm for the rest of humanity, past and present. Experimental evidence from National Institutes of Health research published by Thomas Wehr (1992) could be consistent with a human tendency toward polyphasic sleep. Human subjects were kept in bed in the dark during the evening and nighttime for 14 hours. They demonstrated a sleep pattern consisting of two major sleep episodes separated by middle-of-the-night wakeful periods of one to three hours.

The cultural relativity of sleep schedule norms readily is apparent in the siesta example. In some societies there is an expectation for afternoon napping, even to the extent that businesses are closed at that time. One person's ideal routine of six and one-half hours of nighttime sleep and a 90-minute afternoon nap is another person's day-night cycle of misery, with frustration due to inadequate nighttime sleepiness, insufficient total sleep, and subsequent daytime sleepiness forcing him or her to nap each afternoon.

Summary

The life-story perspective represents explanation based on the logic of the historical narrative. It is a natural, common, and familiar mode of thought, which often is used in clinical situations. Its strengths include the compelling story, which emphasizes the setting and role of the individual, and its potential guidance regarding treatment. The vulnerabilities of this perspective are that the explanations may be poorly testable and can lead to fruitless avenues of therapy.

There always is a broad context with the occurrence of insomnia. The explanation of the sleep disturbance from the sufferer, which perhaps evolves further in a therapeutic relationship, typically involves a time-based narrative highlighting the sequence of contributing factors and the resulting poor sleep outcome. Insomnia becomes the understandable reaction in the intersection of the individual's disposition and circumstances. The recognition of potential causes (e.g., personality features, bedtime routines, schedules, and use of caffeine) for this person's insomnia at this time can reveal meaningful connections, suggest specific treatment strategies, and offer hope for improvement. Specific behavior changes, improvements in sleep hygiene, and psychotherapy goals may be individualized and ultimately may involve a change in the insomnia story.

Groups of insomnia sufferers also may benefit from explanation derived from the life-story perspective, as it provides the foundation of three leading general models of chronic insomnia theory and management: sleep restriction, stimulus control, and cognitive-behavioral therapy. Additionally, a widely used, overarching temporal framework of factors that may contribute to the predisposition, precipitation, and perpetuation of insomnia is based on this mode of reasoning.

An individual's cultural context may strongly influence his or her vulnerability, explanation, and treatment strategies for sleep disturbances. Cross-cultural considerations emphasize the tremendous diversity in the human sleep environment and experience and ultimately may question the ethnocentricity of what in industrial Western societies is called insomnia.

6

Insomnia as a Symptom or a Disease

Insomnia is a common symptom resulting from many disease processes.

The Disease Perspective

The attribution of illness to an abnormality in the structure or function of a bodily part is essential to disease reasoning. The disease model perspective assumes that people share certain illness symptoms, signs, and clinical course characteristics because they share the same underlying physical problem. Clearly, this type of reasoning represents the backbone of contemporary medical science and clinical practice.

The disease model ultimately is a stepwise process; it begins with observing, then categorizing findings, and finally explaining clinical phenomena. Similar clinical presentations, including the course, signs, and symptoms, may be described as syndromes. This should stimulate attempts at explanation, typically through the recognition of similar underlying pathological conditions. The ultimate goal is the identification of one or more specific etiological processes responsible for the pathology.

McHugh and Slavney (1998) emphasize this relationship of the clinical syndrome, pathological process, and etiology. They offer congestive heart failure as an example of a general medical syndrome, which has several potential types of associated pathology, including myocardial infarction, valvular stenosis, hyperthyroidism, and constriction of the pericardial lining. Constrictive pericarditis, in turn, may have the specific etiology of a tubercular infection.

In the realm of psychiatry, dementia is a well-defined syndrome characterized by a global decline in mental functioning. Dementia is a clinical diagnosis based on psychological features and the course of the symptoms. However, various pathological processes can lead to the typical presentation of dementia. Alzheimer disease, multiple infarcts, severe major depression, and pernicious anemia are among the possible underlying pathological entities. Vitamin B_{12} deficiency may be the etiology of the pernicious anemia, just as a genetic defect may be established as the cause of Alzheimer disease.

Schizophrenia also may be viewed as a syndrome with characteristic positive and negative symptoms and, generally, a chronic course. However, there often is considerable variation in the clinical presentation. The range of patients diagnosable with this disorder makes it a rather disjunctive syndrome category. Some have suggested that schizophrenia is best considered as a group of disorders. Of course, evidence of definitive pathology would help greatly in diagnosing psychotic patients. While various avenues of investigation, such as neuroimaging and pharmacological studies, are very promising, pathological processes and etiological agents are not yet firmly proclaimed. The current state of our science, however, does not disqualify schizophrenia from the disease model; we simply remain frustrated at the syndrome level. Ultimately, new data will promote new categorization and explanation and, it is hoped, new treatment approaches.

The disease model has enormous strength and value. It is a familiar mode of thought; the inherent formation and testing of a scientific hypothesis typically is automatic in clinical practice. This approach promotes the accumulation of knowledge that helps explain not just pathology but also normal functioning. The effective recognition of causes leads to rational treatments and preventive measures. However, the disease perspective does deemphasize the role of individuals and their unique vulnerabilities in contributing to their clinical presentations. Further, there is a risk of overapplication of disease reasoning. McHugh and Slavney warn against the potential imperialism of assuming brain pathology for all mental symptoms. They note that some features, such as emotional responses and temperament, are better appreciated with alternative explanatory models.

The Disease Model and Insomnia

In the realm of disease model reasoning, language is very important. Certain precision is inherent in the model for the use of words such as *disease*, *syndrome,* and *symptom.* However, especially with the word *disease,* casual use often is rather vague and may be synonymous with the general notions of disorder or illness. In the disease model, the assumption of physical pathology and the potential for unambiguous etiology always is implied. Where, then, does the word *insomnia* fit into the disease model? The word *insomnia,* without further elaboration, is remarkably imprecise. This is an advantage, since the idea of insomnia is quite broad. But the use of the word alone reveals little to help with a differential diagnosis.

> **The Surprised Insomniac:** May was a 75-year-old woman who came to the Sleep Disorders Center accompanied by her husband. She fretfully described her long history of difficulty falling asleep, periods of sleeplessness during the night, and early morning awakening, as well as how terrible she felt during the daytime. As the sleep specialist reviewed the details of her insomnia complaints with her, she suddenly grasped her husband's arm and, in a surprised and distressed manner, stated, "Oh, my God, then I must have insomnia."

May had avoided the dreaded word *insomnia* in offering her lengthy description of her sleeplessness. To her, an imagined diagnosis called insomnia must have been almost like cancer. Her usage implied that she worried about having some terrible disease called insomnia. Obviously the meaning of *insomnia* for patients and practitioners should be clear. Only then can an effective formulation and treatment plan be developed. For any clinical presentation of insomnia, disease model reasoning will involve information gathering, hypothesis testing, and at least a tentative conclusion as to whether the individual's insomnia complaint does, in fact, represent a diagnosis. Generally, the disease approach has great potential value with insomnia, since it guides classification, stimulates research, and targets management strategies and prevention. Implicit in the model is that it may explain insomnia in certain circumstances.

In chapter 1, insomnia was defined most generally as the complaint of suffering due to not being able to sleep when one wants to sleep. In this very broad sense, then, insomnia simply is a complaint. In certain circumstances, insomnia may be an understandable reaction. For instance, someone might receive a telephone call with distressing news shortly before bedtime and then have great difficulty falling asleep that night. It is not necessary to medicalize this reaction with disease reasoning. In other circumstances, however, insomnia may be regarded as a symptom of a recognized disorder (e.g., medical, psychiatric, or primary sleep disorder). In this regard, insomnia may be seen as a feature contributing to the definition of a syndrome (e.g., major depression), which, in turn, may have its own recognized underlying pathology and etiology.

The disease model stimulates this three-part question: Can insomnia be its own syndrome? If so, can there be identifiable pathology causing the sleep disturbance, and is it possible to confirm an etiological process? The ultimate question becomes, Is there an insomnia disease? The extent to which the disease model is applicable to the complaint of insomnia is explored through the remainder of this chapter with the consideration of insomnia representing a complaint, symptom, syndrome, pathological process, and disease.

The Complaint Insomnia

Insomnia always is a complaint, no matter what else it may be. Insomnia often may be understood as a reaction to particular circumstances and therefore, may be appreciated best with the life-story perspective. Individual vulnerability for experiencing insomnia is emphasized with the dimensional perspective. A brief and reactive insomnia, perhaps from excitement, distress, or worry, may not meet the threshold of bringing the complaint to a health care provider, although this action alone does not reflect severity or chronicity, as many insomnia sufferers do not seek treatment. Sometimes insomnia is just insomnia, and it need not be forced into the disease model. The reactive sleepless experience may not represent a symptom, syndrome, or disease. That is not to say it should be ignored, as healthy habits, behavior changes, stress reduction, or psychotherapy might prove beneficial.

Jet lag and shift work schedules may be associated with insomnia, which may be profound and result in severe consequences. These disturbances are explainable, are reasonably diagnosable, and potentially are treatable. There is a clear physiological connection with the intrinsic circadian system, which anatomically is associated with the suprachiasmatic nucleus. Disease model reasoning would seem obvious here, were it not for the fact that in these cases the *normal* circadian physiology is causing the adverse sleep-wake cycle disturbance, and therefore there is no proposed pathology to support a syndrome, much less a disease. Behavior is the culprit, and the motivated behavior perspective provides the best explanation.

The Symptom Insomnia

Most contemporary educational programs on insomnia begin by emphasizing that it is a symptom and not a disease. For present, perhaps fastidious, purposes, it is argued that insomnia sometimes is not truly a symptom either. Nevertheless, it is useful to highlight the multitude of possible causes of insomnia and that it should be appreciated in a broad clinical context. As a symptom, insomnia may be the chief complaint or an accompanying problem resulting from an underlying medical, psychiatric, substance abuse, or sleep disorder. Resolving the insomnia symptom often requires treating the primary problem.

Various patterns of sleep disruption predictably may result from certain medical disorders, and sometimes insomnia is part of a constellation of symptoms constituting a particular medical syndrome. The life-story perspective highlights the reactive element, as with anxiety regarding worsening health and being given a medical diagnosis. The disease perspective offers explanation where there is abnormal physiology or anatomy directly influencing sleep. A comprehensive review would be encyclopedic, but a few examples are offered here. Hyperthyroidism, in promoting excessive stimulation, undermines sleep, thereby causing the symptom of insomnia. Orthopnea, nocturia, and recurrent gastroesophageal reflux all can promote nighttime awakenings. Chronic obstructive pulmonary disease and congestive heart disease commonly are associated with difficulty maintaining sleep. Any medical disorder causing acute or chronic pain or any significant discomfort may make achieving sufficient sleep rather challenging. Patients diagnosed with fibromyalgia almost invariably report insomnia, and sleep disturbance is included in the diagnostic criteria for chronic fatigue syndrome. Underlying medical illness obviously plays a role in the following case.

> *Altitude Insomnia:* A 72-year-old theoretical physicist presented to the Sleep Disorders Center because of concerns about intermittent insomnia that had impaired his daytime functioning during the past few years. He had mild congestive heart failure, which was relatively well controlled.

He reported that he slept reasonably well while staying at his home near sea level. Several times a year he made extended trips to Los Alamos, New Mexico (elevation over 4,200 feet), and this predictably was when his insomnia occurred. Ultimately, he found that using nasal oxygen at the high altitude allowed much-improved sleep.

Altitude insomnia occurs with everyone at a very high altitude due to the effects of low atmospheric pressure on pulmonary physiology. This patient's insomnia occurred at a moderately high altitude because of this process in conjunction with his congestive heart failure. Both obesity and pregnancy may result in compromised respiration during sleep, ultimately resulting in recurrent awakenings. In the case of pregnancy, hormonal changes and, by the last trimester, physical discomfort also may interfere with sleep.

As with medical disorders, insomnia resulting from psychiatric illnesses may have direct and indirect determinants. The distress and demoralization of having a psychiatric illness may be exacerbated further by the affective, anxiety, or even psychotic features of the disorder. Of particular interest regarding the disease model and insomnia is the potential for physiological processes directly influencing aspects of sleep regulation. Insomnia may be associated with any psychiatric process, but it is most clearly identified as a symptom in the mood disorders and anxiety disorders; however, some evidence suggests sleep deterioration in schizophrenia, as well. Issues of insomnia and excessive sleepiness among psychiatric patients are complicated further by the stimulating or sedating effects of many psychotropic medications.

Major depression is the classic example of a psychiatric disorder causing insomnia, which then generally improves with the resolution of the depression. There is very strong epidemiological evidence supporting the association between major depression and insomnia, and various avenues of research have documented alterations in sleep architecture and other electrophysiological measures in patients with major depression (Perlis et al., 1997). By definition, insomnia is a symptom of major depression: the *Diagnostic and Statistical Manual of Mental Disorders* (DSM-IV) defines the major depression syndrome with criteria requiring the presence of various features of clinical history and symptoms, one option being sleep disturbance (most commonly insomnia but possibly hypersomnolence). The vast majority of patients experiencing major depressive episodes will report significant problems with sleep, which may involve difficulty falling asleep and maintaining sleep, early morning awakening, or any combination of these. Accompanying these subjective complaints are characteristic electrophysiological changes.

Polysomnographic studies of patients with major depression demonstrate a deterioration of sleep continuity, as evidenced by prolonged sleep-onset latency, multiple arousals and awakenings, and poor sleep efficiency. There also tends to be a significant decrease and a characteristic redistribution of slow-wave sleep. Most specific are changes with rapid eye movement (REM) sleep, which often include a shortened latency to the first REM episode and a general redistribution of REM activity toward the early part of the night. Although the percentage of REM sleep may not change, there does tend to be a greater density of eye movements when the depressed person is in REM sleep. Research investigations, including family studies, continue to explore the question of these changes in sleep architecture and the degree to which they may represent state versus trait markers of major depression (Giles et al., 1998).

> *Depressed and Not Sleeping:* Frances was a 76-year-old woman who presented to the Sleep Disorders Center along with her husband because of her complaints of insomnia and a markedly disrupted sleep-wake schedule during the previous year. Before that, she had usually slept well between 11:00 P.M. and 7:00 A.M., but more recently she had been sleeping much less and spending much more time in bed. By late afternoon she would look forward to retiring to bed, and often she went to bed by 9:00 P.M. It would take her many hours to fall asleep. She estimated getting only one to two hours of sleep most nights. She always would be awake for the day by 4:00 A.M., but she remained in bed at least until 9:00 A.M. Typically she would go out briefly and then return home for lunch around noon. She then would return to bed and sleep for up to two hours. She also described feeling depressed during the past year. She had lost interest in her usual activities, and she felt more withdrawn and isolative. She had also experienced a decrease in her appetite, energy, and concentration.

Frances easily was diagnosed with major depression. The difficulty with her sleep probably was influenced directly by the mood disorder; however, her profound withdrawal seemed to promote her excessive time in bed, which further undermined her circadian system, thereby making consolidated sleep less achievable. She responded well with a treatment plan that incorporated antidepressant medication and behavioral changes that focused on her daytime activities.

Although subjective sleep changes very often accompany manic episodes, the report of insomnia is less valuable as a symptom in patients with bipolar disorder. During manic episodes, the total daily sleep amount frequently is reduced, sometimes quite dramatically; however, the manic patient typically is not attempting to sleep and, therefore, is not complaining of insomnia. Nevertheless, some patients experiencing hypomanic or manic episodes will be frustrated by their episode-associated inability to sleep and subsequently will report insomnia as a symptom. Bipolar patients with depressive episodes also commonly suffer from sleep disturbance, most often insomnia and occasionally hypersomnolence.

> *The Manic Insomniac:* A 63-year-old woman diagnosed with bipolar disorder and treated with mood stabilizers complained of increasing difficulty with her sleep over a three-week period. Generally, she had been sleeping well during recent years, but now she had great difficulty both initiating and maintaining sleep. She was extremely frustrated, and she estimated that she got only one to two hours of sleep each night. Uncharacteristically, she became quite demanding about medications, and she began calling every possible psychiatrist and therapist with whom she had had contact over the previous 20 years to discuss her sleep problem. Ultimately, her complaints included bizarre and delusional content. She was assessed as experiencing a manic exacerbation of her bipolar disorder.

A natural question is what physiological process inherent in mood disorders drives the subjectively reported and objectively measured sleep deterioration common in these syndromes: Where is the pathology of affective-related insomnia? There are many clues in the parallel regulation of mood and sleep. Robert McCarley (1982) elegantly reviewed this intersection of mood and sleep in the context of the monoaminergic-cholinergic balance. We assume that important elements of the pathology of mood disorders depend on the neurotransmitter and receptor activities of norepinephrine, serotonin, and dopamine, and it is likely that sleep pathology in depression is associated with this neurotransmitter arena as well. As for the etiology of mood disorders, genetics must be a major factor, but the ultimate answers await further discovery.

The symptom of anxiety frequently is accompanied by sleeplessness; in fact, often it is an expected consequence. As with the mood disorders, direct and indirect influences are likely, but anxiety and insomnia may be more challenging to disentangle. Sleep disturbance may be a symptom of primary anxiety disorders, including generalized anxiety disorder, panic disorder, obsessive-compulsive disorder, and posttraumatic stress disorder. As with the mood disorders, the pathology probably rests with neurotransmitters and the etiology is not firmly established.

Patients diagnosed with panic disorder very often complain of insomnia; however, it is not included in the DSM-IV diagnostic criteria. Additionally, many patients with panic disorder experience extremely distressing panic attacks emanating from sleep, and a few seem to have panic attacks only during sleep. The fear of these nocturnal events secondarily can increase bedtime anxiety and exacerbate the insomnia.

> *Panic Awakenings:* Andrew was a 37-year-old, married man employed as a systems analyst for a governmental agency. His evaluation at the Sleep Disorders Center was prompted by the worsening of his sleep disturbance, which had begun about five years previously. He felt that his sleep difficulties were interfering with his daytime work performance. During this period he had experienced sudden awakenings within an hour of sleep onset. He described a sense of being "jerked out of sleep" by these events that were associated with tachycardia, tachypnea, and diaphoresis. He would have to sit on the side of the bed and wait for his intense anxiety to subside. Previously, these events had occurred just a few times a year, but now it was happening almost weekly. Furthermore, over the past year he had felt anxious as bedtime approached, and most nights he experienced significant difficulty falling asleep.

Insomnia formally is considered a common element of the generalized anxiety disorder syndrome, as the DSM-IV criteria include the option of associated "sleep disturbance (difficulty falling or staying asleep, or restless unsatisfying sleep)." Certainly, there is considerable phenomenological overlap between the general constant worrier and the constant worrier about sleep.

> *Racing-Mind Insomnia:* Janet was a 38-year-old homemaker when her primary care physician suggested her Sleep Disorders Center evaluation for longstanding complaints of difficulty sleeping. She had been in outpatient psychiatric treatment continuously for seven years and intermittently for nine years before that. She had been diagnosed with generalized anxiety disorder, and along with psychotherapy and relaxation training,

she had been prescribed many different antidepressants and anxiolytics. Over the past year, her only medication had been fluoxetine. She described feeling anxious throughout the daytime but noted that her anxiety seemed worse in the late evening as bedtime approached. She felt somewhat sleepy in the evening, but when she would get in bed about 11:30 P.M. she felt that her mind was racing. She described worrying about everything imaginable, such as the previous day's events, financial concerns, family affairs, her future health, and world peace. She would remain sleepless in bed for one to two hours before falling into a light sleep. She had the sense that any sort of noise or other external disturbance would immediately awaken her, at which time her mind would "switch into high gear." Often she was awake before hearing her 7:00 A.M. alarm. Although she typically felt fatigued during the daytime, she never felt sleepy. Overall, she felt that her anxiety symptoms were much improved compared with previous years but that her sleep problems remained just as bad.

Patients with obsessive-compulsive disorder (OCD) typically do not complain of insomnia, except when they are unable to sleep in obvious connection with their obsessive thoughts and compulsive behaviors. Some patients will ruminate uncontrollably when they get in bed, and others will feel compelled to get up and check their alarm clocks, door locks, and other household safety items. One patient of the Sleep Disorders Center who was being treated for OCD described his nightly routine of getting into bed, turning out the lights, and immediately focusing his attention on some event from the previous day. He felt compelled to replay the situation in great detail over and over in his mind. Curiously, polysomnographic studies of obsessive-compulsive patients do suggest some alterations in sleep architecture similar to those found with major depression. This parallel may offer some insight into the pathology of both disorders.

The DSM-IV includes "difficulty falling or staying asleep" among the options in the criteria for posttraumatic stress disorder (PTSD). Insomnia and awakenings from vivid dreams and nightmares are symptoms that follow the trauma in the majority of patients diagnosed with PTSD. Several studies have suggested fundamental abnormalities in REM sleep; however, a preponderance of evidence has not demonstrated a predictable change in sleep architecture.

Explosive Awakenings: Frank was a 46-year-old, married factory worker on disability at the time of his evaluation at the Sleep Disorders Center.

He had been referred from his Regional Burn Center treatment team because of his severely disrupted nighttime sleep. He gave a history of always sleeping well before his injury 10 months previously. He had worked in a factory that produced food ingredients. An explosion at work resulted in second- and third-degree burns to 25 percent of his body, including his arms, neck, chest, and abdomen. He spent about one month on the Burn Unit, and he had had several skin grafts. His wounds had healed appropriately, and he continued with physical therapy and participation in a burn support group. He was hopeful about returning to work, initially on a part-time basis. However, he felt that his progress was limited by his sleep difficulties and daytime fatigue.

Pain and discomfort had made sleep difficult during the few months after the accident, but now that seemed less of a problem. He reported that for the past few months he would feel rather anxious as his 11:00 P.M. bedtime approached, and he started staying up later at night to avoid going to bed. He had difficulty falling asleep, as he dreaded the experiences that he feared awaited him each night. While his sleep always seemed light, it was interrupted at least once, and sometimes two or three times, by terrifying awakenings when he felt that he was reliving the explosion. Often he would scream and jump from his bed. He felt that his heart was pounding and racing. Typically, he would remain awake for about an hour before he was able to return to sleep. He was unable to sleep past 6:00 A.M., and he would get up at that time, even though he did not feel refreshed. During the daytime he tried to remain busy. He said that he felt too "wired" to even think of napping. While he did want to work again and he was motivated to return to his former workplace because of his long-term employment with the company, he was worried about seeing the accident over and over again in his mind when he returned to the factory.

Like many patients diagnosed with PTSD, Frank developed distressing insomnia symptoms, especially the awakenings with vivid images of the explosion and the sense of terror. Ultimately, this sleep disturbance contributed to his ongoing impairment.

Insomnia, particularly sleep-onset difficulty, occurs commonly among patients with schizophrenia, although it is not a specific symptom contributing to the definition of the disorder. The inability to sleep may be severe at times, especially with the exacerbation of psychotic symptoms. Van Kammen et al. (1986) suggest that sleep deterioration may be prodromal to worsening of the primary psychotic features. No clear pathology accounts for this sleep-onset difficulty. However, the electrophysiological characteristics of sleep in schizophrenic persons have been a major research area. Several studies have demonstrated a general deficit of slow-wave sleep among schizophrenic patients, as well as a reduced REM latency; however, neither of these patterns nor an underlying cause is firmly established. Occasionally, patients diagnosed with schizophrenia will report the ultimate insomnia: an absolute inability to sleep for long periods of time.

Sleepless in Schizophrenia: James was a 25-year-old man who, four years previously, had acutely developed pronounced hallucinations and delusions, which led to a series of psychiatric hospitalizations and a diagnosis of schizophrenia. He had been an excellent student and had been doing well in college when the psychotic symptoms began. Ultimately, he was functioning reasonably well, although he was refusing to take any medications. He was successful in pursuing a variety of evaluations by different medical specialists for two complaints that seemed to dominate his life: he claimed that he had lost his memory and his ability to sleep. Regarding his memory, he was able to recite in detail exactly what he claimed to be unable to remember. On further questioning, he described that they no longer felt like memories. He used the analogy of things from the past now being in black and white, when before he experienced them in color. On the topic of sleep, he claimed that it had been more than one year since he had had a single moment of sleep. Household informants confirmed that he seemed to sleep deeply a normal length of time and that often he snored. Typically, during the daytime he was fully alert, and he demonstrated no evidence of sleep insufficiency.

It is tempting to formulate the complaint of complete sleeplessness of some schizophrenic patients as delusional; however, this belief raises the question of the perception of sleep, which to a lesser degree is abnormal in many patients with chronic insomnia. Perhaps, just as the classic phenomenological split of the affective and cognitive realms in schizophrenia may relate to the above patient's complaint of memory loss, there also may be some major defect in the ability to experience the effects of sleep.

Insomnia may be the only complaint or one of many associated with underlying primary sleep disorders. Patients may present to a health care provider or a sleep disorders center with the sole complaint of insomnia and ultimately be diagnosed with sleep-disordered breathing, restless legs syndrome, periodic limb movement disorder, or even one of the parasomnias.

Sleep-disordered breathing involves recurrent apneic (complete breathing cessation) or hypopneic (reduced airflow) episodes due to central or obstructive mechanisms. The events may cause arousals and awakenings in people completely unaware of the breathing disruption. Although the majority of patients with sleep-disordered breathing will complain primarily of excessive sleepiness, insomnia is not an unusual symptom. It typically improves with effective treatment of the sleep-related breathing disruption through continuous positive airway pressure (CPAP), surgery, weight loss, dental appliances, or other means.

Insomnia Central: Paul was a 68-year-old, married man who presented to the Sleep Disorders Center complaining that, although he had slept rather well throughout his life, he has had severe difficulty initiating and maintaining sleep for the past five months. His medical history included a myocardial infarction 10 years previously and a mild stroke 1 year before the sleep center evaluation. The complaint of severe insomnia began with a hospitalization that had been unsuccessful in achieving cardioversion for his atrial fibrillation. He would attempt sleep at his usual bedtime of 11:30 P.M. but typically would not fall asleep until at least 4:00 A.M. He felt quite frustrated, and often he would pace during the night. He estimated that he would get only two or three hours of sleep each night. His wife noted that he appeared rather restless during his limited periods of sleep. His attempts to achieve improved sleep included such strategies as drinking three martinis, undergoing professional hypnosis, and taking various prescribed hypnotics, including chloral hydrate and flurazepam. A polysomnographic study performed after he had discontinued alcohol and hypnotics for several weeks demonstrated that, out of seven and one-half hours in bed, he slept only two hours and that this limited sleep was mostly stage 1. During his sleep he demonstrated recurrent central apneic events (30 per hour) in a Cheyne-Stokes respiration pattern, which is one manifestation of central sleep apnea.

Obstructive sleep apnea is considerably more common than apnea of central origin. Although it is most commonly found in overweight male patients, severe cases may be identified in slender individuals of both sexes. Occasionally, insomnia is the only presenting symptom, and patients are quite surprised with the ultimate diagnosis.

Gasping Insomnia: Larry was 41 years old and married at the time of his evaluation in the Sleep Disorders Center. Previously, he had slept well, but over the past year he had experienced almost hourly awakenings during the night. Often he would awaken and find himself sitting up at the side of the bed. His wife noted his loud snoring and gasping during the night. They both described the profound daytime sleepiness that had been increasing during this time. He now was limiting his driving because of drowsiness. He had gained 130 pounds over the previous year, taking him up to 375 pounds. The obesity was attributed to pituitary damage from an ocular mucocele diagnosed 10 years previously. He was hoping to find a way to sleep through the night and be fully alert during the daytime. A polysomnographic study confirmed the suspected obstructive sleep apnea. His nighttime sleep and daytime alertness were much improved after the initiation of CPAP.

Restless legs syndrome (RLS) frequently is associated with sleep-onset difficulty and sometimes with recurrent nighttime awakenings. Accordingly, insomnia is a very common complaint among RLS patients. RLS is a chronic and progressive condition producing a very disconcerting sensory experience described as restlessness or a creepy-crawly feeling that makes the sufferer want to move the limbs or even pace to relieve the discomfort. Although the sensation is mostly in the legs, it may generalize to other body parts. Twitching may accompany the restlessness. A circadian process seems to influence the timing of the symptoms, as the sensations worsen while one is at rest in the evening as bedtime approaches; however, the restlessness tends to begin earlier in the evening or daytime as the disorder progresses. Evidence points to abnormal central nervous system (CNS) dopamine functioning, and dopaminergic medications often are beneficial. While several causes, including a genetic component, may lead to this syndrome, one is clear: low iron stores. A low ferritin level is associated with an increased risk of RLS symptoms, which in these cases usually will improve with iron supplementation.

The Restless Legs Insomniac: A 45-year-old, married, Arab woman living in a Persian Gulf country came to the medical center for an extensive evaluation. She requested to be seen in the Sleep Disorders Center because of her great distress from insomnia symptoms, which had begun while she was in her mid-20s. She had had an initial episode during her first pregnancy, and then the symptoms resolved. The insomnia returned with the next pregnancy and lasted longer. After her fourth and final pregnancy, five years before the evaluation, the insomnia became persistent. She suffered primarily from sleep-onset difficulty, and she came to dread the evening hours as she anticipated misery. Most nights she would pace and involve herself in various household activities before attempting sleep, which was several hours after the rest of the family had gone to bed. Even 20 years earlier she had associated her insomnia with a sense of restlessness felt most intensely in her legs. Because of the clinical history consistent with RLS, a ferritin level was checked and the value was an extremely low 5 mcg/L.

Pregnancy and anemia have been recognized as risk factors for RLS symptoms in vulnerable individuals. Accordingly, it has been hypothesized that redistribution of iron stores during pregnancy may be the key factor increasing the RLS at that time. With the above patient, there probably was increasing anemia with each pregnancy, and this was compounded by dietary iron deficiency. The very low ferritin level indicated low iron stores and, therefore, high risk.

Periodic limb movements in sleep (PLMS) occur in the majority of RLS patients and in others idiopathically. During sleep and sometimes during waking periods, people with this disorder will experience recurrent brief muscle contractions expressed as leg jerks and sometimes more generally involving the arms or the total body. These events may have no clinical significance; however, when the frequency is high and many of them are associated with electroencephalogram (EEG)-defined arousals, there is greater potential for sleep disruption, which can be rather dramatic for some patients. Sufferers sometimes are unaware of the frequent jerking experiences during their sleep, and they may be aware only of the insomnia and daytime consequences.

Leg Kicks: Jean was a 61-year-old, married woman who presented to the Sleep Disorders Center because of severe disruption of her sleep during the previous three years. She had had no prior difficulty with her sleep but now felt that, without medicine, she was able to get only about three hours of very light sleep each night. She had difficulty falling asleep, but then she could not sleep continuously for more than about 20 minutes. Her husband noted that recently she had been kicking her legs in her sleep. One year previously, while hospitalized, she had been prescribed triazolam, and she continued taking it most nights with moderate benefit. Her medical history included worsening renal insufficiency over the past few years leading to a blood urea nitrogen (BUN) of 80 mg/dL and a creatinine of 5.1 mg/dL. Polysomnographic evaluation showed extremely poor sleep efficiency and a rate of periodic limb movements in the severe range.

The parasomnias represent a very curious array of behaviors and other disturbances emanating from sleep, and several of these may include insomnia as a prominent symptom—and sometimes as the only complaint. Some parasomnias specifically are related to non-REM (NREM) or REM sleep, and others are less specific. The frequency can range from rare to nightly, and the degree of disturbance from benign to dramatic. Typically associated with NREM sleep, especially slow-wave sleep, are sleep terrors, sleepwalking, and confusional arousals. Although it is common for the individual to have no recollection of the events, sometimes complete, and occasionally distressing, awakenings will occur. There may be pronounced autonomic stimulation and difficulty returning to sleep.

The Bomb Scare: Seth was a married, 29-year-old sales representative when he sought help at the Sleep Disorders Center because of his frequent and dramatic nighttime awakenings. His parents told him that as a child he had often sleepwalked and sometimes screamed in his sleep. His sleep was calm through his teen years, but in his early 20s he occasionally began to exhibit rather dramatic behaviors about one hour after falling asleep. Often he awakened fully with a great sense of terror after sitting up and screaming loudly, and occasionally he would leap from his bed and struggle with household objects. On one occasion he tore apart and destroyed a large bedroom houseplant that he thought was an intruder. For a few years the events seemed to occur episodically; there might be several in one week and then none for a few months. After an initial evaluation, he was able to avoid situations that resulted sleep deprivation, and the sleep-related behaviors were rare. He returned to the clinic a few months after the birth of his first child because of a marked increase in the frequency and intensity of the fearful arousals. Soon after the baby was born, he again was suddenly sitting up, screaming, and sometimes bolting from the bed. Occasionally, he returned to sleep with little memory of the event, but usually he awakened fully with an intense sense of terror. On two recent occasions he had been convinced that a bomb was in the house, and he had raced to the baby's room, picked her up, and run down the steps and out of the house. Only then had he fully awakened and appreciated the actual situation. He and his wife had great safety concerns regarding these irrational nighttime behaviors. For several months he took clonazepam, 0.5 mg nightly, and this was successful in eliminating the behaviors and awakenings.

In people who are vulnerable, these sleep terror events seem to occur more frequently during periods of increased stress and insufficient sleep.

For instance, a medical student seen at the center experienced his sleep terrors at a greater rate during exam weeks, when he had more stress and less sleep. In Seth's case, the patient had new worries of financial responsibility after the baby was born, and his sleep-wake schedule had been disrupted by the baby's irregular schedule.

Sleep-related eating is a type of parasomnia in which individuals, after initially sleeping, will get out of bed and compulsively seek out and eat food. Some with this disorder will have no memory of the behavior; others will recall the eating, but feel unable to control it. For many sufferers, the episodes occur nightly and usually relatively early in the night. Witnesses often say the person seems to be sleepwalking. Typically there are not daytime manifestations of traditional eating disorders.

The Sleep-Related Eater: Laura was a 36-year-old woman who came to the Sleep Disorders Center seeking help for her insomnia, which had persisted for 18 years. She stated that her sleep was interrupted every night and that she felt fatigued and sleepy during the daytime. On further questioning, she admitted to an intractable pattern of arising every night, at least once, beginning about one hour after sleep onset. She would go directly to the kitchen and eat. Her food choices, unlike her daytime eating, were for high-fat and high-calorie items, especially with a thick consistency, such as ice cream and peanut butter. Sometimes she felt awake but unable to stop the eating behavior. Other times she knew of the eating because of crumbs and missing food. She always felt full in the morning, and she never ate breakfast. To maintain her normal weight, she mildly restricted her daytime eating, since she knew that she could not stop the eating she would do in her sleep. She had tried various strategies to stop the sleep-related eating, but none had reduced the frequency of the behavior. This included hiding food, putting furniture in the hallway to impede her passage and wake her up, and locking her bedroom door. When she recruited her husband's help to try to awaken her and dissuade her from eating during the nightly episodes, she became agitated and fought with him to attain food. She described feeling like a very different person whenever she did have awareness of her thoughts and behaviors during the events. She also was embarrassed about the eating and the associated behaviors.

REM sleep parasomnias include awakenings with vivid dreaming and nightmares and REM behavior disorder. Sleep disruption is more prominent with these disorders. Nightmares are a familiar phenomenon that by definition involve an awakening and often result in difficulty returning to sleep. Sympathetic stimulation may contribute to the awakenings, especially when there are autonomic symptoms, such as tachycardia and diaphoresis. Frequent nightmares can generate the symptom of chronic insomnia. Anticipation of frequent and distressing nightmares secondarily can promote difficulty falling asleep.

In REM behavior disorder there is faulty disinhibition of the brainstem mechanism that normally prevents the transmission of impulses from the cortical motor areas that are stimulated during dreaming. Those with this disorder will demonstrate motor activity, which may be rather violent and injurious, in conjunction with dreaming in REM sleep. Although there are benign reports of simple movements that are consistent with relatively calm dream content (e.g., swinging an arm while dreaming of playing tennis), most cases involve more intense, and often fearful, dreams. This disorder is more common among elderly persons and may be found in association with various neurological conditions, particularly degenerative disorders. Injurious disruptions of sleep are present in the following case.

Dream Attacks: John was a 65-year-old man seen in the Sleep Disorders Center along with his wife because of his disrupted nighttime sleep. They both stated that for several decades he had been extremely active in his sleep. The problem had worsened over the previous four years. Most nights he would flail, fight, jerk, talk, and scream. Loud cursing was common. Sometimes he would throw objects and fight with furniture. He had hit his wife on several occasions, so they had been sleeping in separate bedrooms for the past four years. They noted one occasion when he was screaming, "I'm finally going to get you." He was standing up holding a blanket and trying to smother his wife. He reported on awakening that he was dreaming about catching his dog. He was distressed about this behavior and was fearful about injuring his wife. Although the events had occurred at all hours of the night, the great majority had been during the last few hours. He noted also that a brother exhibited identical behaviors and that his wife, too, slept in another bedroom.

Various other primary sleep disturbances also may include a strong insomnia component and may be associated with daytime impairment. This is evident in the following case example, where several factors increase the risk for the patient's primary sleep disorder.

Wet Awakenings: Horace was a 24-year-old, married man who presented to the Sleep Disorders Center along with his wife. He sought help because of his nightly awakenings, his difficulty concentrating at work during the daytime, and his embarrassment about his problem. He had been experiencing bedwetting throughout his life. Generally, the enuretic episodes were nightly; however, he had had a few dry periods of up to a few weeks in the past. His sleep would be disturbed only after he felt cold and wet. He was unsure of any factors that might exacerbate or alleviate the bedwetting. His typical schedule included a 1:00 A.M. bedtime, a 6:00 A.M. awakening for work, and a 6:00 P.M. nap. To help stay awake and alert during the daytime, he drank about two pots of coffee throughout the daytime and up until bedtime.

As disease model reasoning emphasizes the pathology that may underlie the insomnia experience, this approach is useful in considering the potential influence of medications on sleep. Obviously, a great many medications may have direct stimulating effects or indirect actions (e.g., diuretics) that can undermine efficient sleep. The following individual viewed himself as requiring long-term use of hypnotic medication for his presumed chronic insomnia.

> *Withdrawal Insomnia:* Peter was a 50-year-old, married computer programmer when he was referred to the Sleep Disorders Center for insomnia that had begun suddenly 10 years previously. At that time he had been undergoing a divorce from his first wife. He had found this process to be quite stressful, and he had begun taking a benzodiazepine hypnotic at that time. Without taking medication for sleep, he felt that it had been taking him several hours to fall asleep, but with the hypnotic, he was able to go to bed at about 11:00 P.M., fall asleep within 30 minutes, and then sleep soundly until about 7:00 A.M. Generally, he felt alert during the daytime. On several occasions during the previous decade, he decided to discontinue the hypnotic medication. Usually, this was when a prescription ran out, and he thought he no longer would require the pill for help with sleep. On each occasion his sleep was terrible for several nights, and he would frantically call his physician for another prescription. He finally felt convinced that he had a serious problem, since he seemed unable to sleep without the medication. He wondered whether further testing should be done to discover what was wrong with him.

The withdrawal insomnia experienced by this patient after his abrupt discontinuation of the traditional benzodiazepine hypnotic after long-term use was not surprising. Unfortunately, it led to the strengthening of his conclusion that he required the chronic use of the medication for his sleep to be satisfactory. Ultimately, a very gradual reduction of the hypnotic, along with education and support through follow-up visits, was helpful in achieving the goal of good sleep without the medication. Fortunately, newer generation hypnotics are much less likely to promote withdrawal effects and therefore do not tend to promote indefinite use in this manner.

Insomnia Syndromes

Thus far, with insomnia, either the disease model perspective is not applicable because there is no suspicion of an abnormal bodily structure or function causing the sleep disturbance, or the insomnia is seen as a symptom of another disorder where a physical cause is suspected. The question now is whether there is a primary type of insomnia, not due to another disorder, that might be considered as its own syndrome. This idea of an independent insomnia is supported by the current major sleep nosologies, as noted in chapter 1. The DSM-IV incorporates a diagnosis called primary insomnia. The *International Classification of Sleep Disorders Diagnostic and Coding Manual* (ICSD) defines three categories of chronic insomnia complainers in whom an intrinsic process is assumed: psychophysiological insomnia, idiopathic insomnia, and sleep-state misperception. All four of these diagnoses inherently are syndromes, and all are rather broad in scope and inclusion. Only the diagnosis of psychophysiological insomnia presumes any pathology, in this case psychological in nature. Accordingly, those individuals meeting the rather general criteria of sleep disturbance with "somatized tension and learned sleep-preventing associations" may be considered as sharing this syndrome of conditioned arousal associated with attempts to sleep (Diagnostic Classification Steering Committee, 1990).

The general notion of insomnia has no real boundary other than the complaint of sleeplessness and, therefore, is too broad to represent a syndrome definition. However, particular populations of insomnia sufferers do share specific features of their clinical courses and patterns of sleep disturbance. In fact, it can be argued that abnormalities in physiological functioning may be causing the sleep difficulties.

Physiological processes must be presumed with patients whose circadian rhythm is disordered, as described in chapter 4, "The Dimensions of Sleep." Objective measurements of the circadian phase, such as the timing of melatonin secretion and core body temperature, also correspond with the subjective sleepiness experience and sleep propensity. The circadian system is unusually early in those with the advanced sleep phase syndrome and is unusually late in those with the delayed sleep phase syndrome. A complete lack of entrainment with the photoperiod, as with blind free-running patients, also has a primary abnormal circadian influence. In all of these disorders, physiological variation from norms is evident, and the afflicted individuals share similar symptoms, clinical courses, and consequences. Therefore, a syndromal designation would be appropriate in these clinical situations.

Insomnia Syndromes with Pathology

The disease model challenges an explanation for observed syndromes. As noted above, large groups of chronic insomnia sufferers are purported to have an idiopathic insomnia that might be termed primary or psychophysiological in nature. These individuals describe a long history of persistent frustration due to their chronic difficulty initiating and maintaining sleep and a sense that the sleep they achieve is very light and never refreshing. Typically, they are anxious, irritable, fatigued, and unable to sleep during the daytime, and they are particularly tense and worried throughout the evening as bedtime approaches. Explanation for this symptom cluster has been sought in the physiological realm in accord with the disease model reasoning. Several hypotheses have been offered using physiological evidence in the attempt to account for both major daytime and nighttime symptoms of patients with this chronic insomnia syndrome.

In a classic 1967 study, Monroe and colleagues measured indicators of physiological arousal in two groups of subjects: individuals reporting that they typically experienced good sleep and those reporting poor sleep. The poor sleep subjects were more physiologically activated both before sleep onset and during sleep, as evidenced by increased heart rate, basal skin resistance, core body temperature, and phasic vasoconstrictions. Monroe found that the subjective report predicted the objective arousal, and he concluded that "self-reported poor sleepers not only sleep less, but the sleep they obtain is more 'awake-like' than that of good sleepers." A hypothesis of pathological physiological activation promoting the typical 24-hour chronic insomnia symptom cluster has evolved with several elaborations. A key question remains: What is the underlying cause of this measurable physiological pathology? It has been suggested that it is due to a fundamental etiology in the physiological realm, perhaps with genetic influence, or, alternatively, that the physiological manifestation results from a psychological source. Anxiety straddles these two realms, so differentiation is rather challenging.

Bonnet and Arand (1997) presented a compelling argument for such a syndrome of chronic insomnia based on the pathology of persistent excessive arousal of the sympathetic nervous system. They emphasized that, for these individuals, insomnia is a 24-hour arousal disorder, and they suggested that this persistent arousal will account for both the nighttime and the daytime experiences of the patients. These symptoms include the perception of insufficient nighttime sleep, as well as daytime irritability, anxiety, tension, fatigue, and inability to sleep during attempts at napping.

In a clever series of studies, Bonnet and Arand monitored true insomniac subjects; a group of artificially hyperaroused normals, who were given caffeine, 400 mg three times a day for one week; and a group of normals who were "yoked" to the actual reduced sleep schedule of insomniac persons for one week. The hyperaroused normals had evidence of physiological activation similar to that of the chronic insomniac persons, and they also had the experience of very poor sleep. The physiological activation included increased metabolic rate and body temperature and decreased daytime sleep propensity, and there was a subjective sense of fatigue and increased anxiety. The authors suggested that the induced hyperarousal promotes psychological changes, such as an elevated anxiety scale on the Minnesota Multiphasic Personality Inventory, in contrast to a hypothesis of primary personality and psychological pathology driving the physiological activation.

The protocol of yoke-controlled normals was developed to determine whether the typical daytime experience for people with chronic insomnia (anxiety, tension, and fatigue) results from persistent insufficient sleep, as most insomnia sufferers believe, or from persistent excessive physiological arousal. The normals were subjected to the objectively measured reduced and interrupted sleep of the chronic insomnia group. This sleep deprivation for the normals resulted in an increased daytime and nighttime sleep propensity obviously not present for the insomnia group sleeping the same total amount. Compared with the chronic insomnia group, during the daytime the yoke-controlled normals had a lower metabolic rate and core body temperature and also lower scores on tension and depression scales. Like the persons with chronic insomnia, these partially sleep-deprived normals did experience an increase in fatigue and a decrease in vigor. Together these findings suggest that persistent hyperarousal promotes the daytime symptoms of chronic insomnia as well as the nighttime experience of insufficient sleep. For individuals with chronic insomnia, this physiological activation counters the effect of partial sleep deprivation, which increases the daytime sleep propensity in normals.

Bonnet and Arand concluded that individuals can be categorized along two independent scales, creating a grid of extreme conditions. The scales represent inherent and enduring characteristics, consistent with dimensional perspective vulnerabilities, which correspond with a low-to-high basal arousal level and with a short-to-long sleep requirement. Typical individuals with chronic insomnia would fall into the combined extremes of high arousal and short sleep requirement, while those at the extremes of high arousal and long sleep requirement would sleep a normal amount but still have the experience of insufficient sleep and daytime fatigue and anxiety. This latter group would account for those individuals diagnosed with sleep state misperception—complaining of chronic insomnia but objectively sleeping a normal duration. The authors believe that effective treatment for the general syndrome of excessively aroused chronic insomnia must be directed toward the entire 24-hour sleep-wake cycle and not simply focused on bedtime strategies—behavioral or pharmacological.

Pathology in the hypothalamic-pituitary-adrenal (HPA) axis is the core of the hypothesis espoused by Vgontzas and colleagues (2001) at the Pennsylvania State University. They argue that chronic insomnia is a disorder of hyperarousal throughout the 24-hour sleep-wake cycle. They point out that the daytime experience and assessments of patients with chronic insomnia (increased perceived stress, anxiety, and depression; increased body temperature, metabolic rate, and heart rate) are very different from those of healthy controls subjected to a similar degree of sleep loss (decreased anxiety, objective and subjective sleepiness). To support the hypothesis that chronic insomnia is caused by dysfunction of the HPA axis, they present data demonstrating significantly elevated levels of plasma adrenocorticotropic hormone (ACTH) and cortisol throughout 24-hour recordings. Subjects with insomnia experienced the greatest sleep disturbance in the evening and first half of the night, which was when the plasma levels showed the greatest elevation. The investigators concluded that chronic insomnia is a disorder of persistent 24-hour CNS hyperarousal, as opposed to a primary problem of sleep loss.

Another explanatory approach to the syndrome of the hyperaroused individual with chronic insomnia focuses on electrophysiological pathology. Michael Perlis and colleagues (2001) argued that the experience of chronic insomnia is associated with abnormal cortical arousal, resulting in altered sensory and cognitive phenomena related to attempts at sleep onset. Agreeing with the widely accepted model of conditioned hyper-arousal in chronic insomnia, Perlis et al. went on to suggest that a high-frequency EEG in the beta and gamma ranges is a key element of the conditioned response.

According to Perlis et al., the presence of this high-frequency EEG activity promotes abnormal increased information processing and corresponding long-term memory formation. Normally, at sleep onset there is a general slowing of the EEG. However, among chronic insomnia sufferers there is evidence of a relative increase in the high-frequency bins before sleep onset and during several minutes into sleep. The hypothesized increased sensory processing would have persons with chronic insomnia being more aware of their environment, and this might cause them to be more likely to interpret their mental state as wakefulness. The normal experience of sleep onset may have an inherent amnesia that is prevented in these insomnia sufferers by their high-frequency EEG-driven cortical arousal. If long-term memory function is enhanced during the peri-sleep-onset phase, then the memory of sleeplessness may promote the interpretation of insomnia. Perlis et al. suggested that this could account for the common overestimation of nighttime wakefulness among individuals with chronic insomnia.

Within this framework of chronic insomnia incorporating a conditioned cortical arousal that influences the experience and memory of wakefulness, the beneficial effects of benzodiazepine-related hypnotics might partially be due to decreased sensory processing and increased amnestic action occurring at sleep onset. Perlis et al. also suggested that this conditioned cortical arousal could explain the subjective experience of insomnia in those individuals objectively found to sleep a normal duration and, therefore, might be given the label of sleep-state misperception.

The Etiology of Insomnia

The ultimate goal when investigating a syndrome with recognized pathology is identification of the etiological agent. Clearly, syndromes of chronic insomnia can be formulated. In some cases, physiological evidence does suggest a realm of pathology. But there is not yet a clearly defined disease of idiopathic insomnia that has an identifiable etiology—that is, the cause of the faulty functioning of a bodily part. However, the science of disease models does encourage speculation.

Emmanuel Mignot (2001) has been instrumental in recent progress regarding the pathophysiology of narcolepsy. For several years it has been evident that the balance of monoaminergic and cholinergic activities influences alertness, sleepiness, REM and NREM sleep, and the potential for cataplexy, which is the sudden muscle weakness that may occur during heightened emotions in narcoleptic patients. In the clinical management of patients with narcolepsy, stimulants have been used to treat the excessive sleepiness, and certain antidepressants (combining assorted monoamine reuptake blockade and anticholinergic activity) have been beneficial in reducing cataplexy. A strong human leukocyte antigen (HLA) locus association (DQB1*0602 and DQA1*0102) also has been established with narcolepsy, especially in those patients with cataplexy. Research with animal models for this most specific type of narcolepsy that includes cataplexy has identified abnormal functioning of the neuropeptide hypocretin system, which in the case of narcoleptic dogs involves faulty receptor encoding due to exon-skipping mutations. It is hypothesized that a hypocretin deficiency promotes dopaminergic hypoactivity and cholinergic hyperactivity, accounting for the sleepiness, cataplexy, and increased REM activity observed with narcolepsy.

With this advancement in understanding the etiology of the sleepiness of narcolepsy, is there any potential insight for the opposite symptom: the sleeplessness of chronic insomnia? Not yet; however, Mignot (2001) conjectured that perhaps the reversed situation—a hypocretin excess—could cause an underlying imbalance in the sleep-wake cycle that makes the experience of sufficient sleep unattainable for some insomnia patients. A neuroanatomical explanation for chronic insomnia that would involve persistently increased monoamine activity is imaginable in this framework. Perhaps someday a genetic defect could be identified as the cause of a specific disease of chronic insomnia, which could allow a specific remedy for what we now must appreciate as a syndrome.

Summary

The disease model perspective represents the foundation of contemporary medical science and clinical practice. The model promotes classification and explanation for symptoms in the realm of pathology—abnormality in the structure or functioning of bodily parts. Syndromes are defined and categorized by constellations of shared symptoms and features of the clinical course. The next step in explanation is identification of the pathology underlying syndromes. Finally, the etiological process causing the pathology may be discovered and elucidated. This disease model process builds on accumulating knowledge, and among the goals is effective treatment.

Most generally, insomnia is a complaint—the inability to sleep when one wants to sleep. Acute or chronic insomnia commonly is a symptom of a medical, psychiatric, or primary sleep disorder. Effective treatment of the underlying disorder may be necessary for a resolution of the insomnia.

Idiopathic types of chronic insomnia may be formulated as syndromes. Included here are the nosological categories of primary insomnia (DSM-IV) and psychophysiological insomnia (ICSD). A chronic insomnia syndromal designation also may be useful with the general group of patients regarded as having a sleep-related conditioned hyperarousal, as well as those individuals suffering with the advanced or delayed sleep phase syndromes.

Physiological parameters have been examined in controls and groups of patients with chronic insomnia including a syndrome of conditioned hyperarousal. The proposed pathology involves excessive sympathetic arousal (decreased sleep propensity, increased metabolic rate and core body temperature) and cortical arousal (increased high-frequency EEG activity). One speculative model of the etiology of sleeplessness in chronic insomnia is based on recent evidence regarding the excessiveness of sleepiness associated with narcolepsy and cataplexy.

7

Evaluation and Treatment

The Need for Integration

The causes of insomnia are multifactorial.

T he global conclusion from the previous chapters on the four perspectives is that the experience and complaint of insomnia result from a
remarkably wide diversity of processes and that the causes of sleeplessness
can be approached with very different explanatory models. Following the
design of McHugh and Slavney's *Perspectives of Psychiatry* (1998), this
book has examined corresponding models of explanation for insomnia.
Accordingly, insomnia has been considered from these four fundamentally
distinct avenues of understanding:

1. Insomnia results from a decreased drive of sleepiness.
2. Insomnia occurs in predisposed individuals because of their enduring vulnerabilities.
3. Insomnia is an understandable response to life circumstances.
4. Insomnia is a common symptom resulting from many disease
   processes.

Now that each has been elaborated, can these explanatory models be
integrated to create a grand schema of insomnia causation? Certainly, a
complex diagram with multiple boxes and arrows could be constructed in
the attempt to connect assorted influences and outcomes. Alternatively, a
lengthy multivariate equation could be concocted to suggest these relationships. However, such efforts would produce rather artificial results, as

these dimensions of explanation do not necessarily intersect. The real answer is that there is no all-encompassing, dimension-transcending, unified conceptualization to fully integrate these explanatory approaches. Each model has its own validity and internal consistency, and each has inherent strengths and weaknesses. However, in no way are the explanatory models mutually exclusive. Fundamentally, the paradigms provide different answers because they raise different questions. The good news is that one need not have to choose the single right one; in fact, attempting to do so often will limit the scope of the clinical appreciation of a case. The more important issue is whether the models are valuable in any particular clinical situation. A comprehensive evaluation of an individual complaining of insomnia will consider potential influences highlighted in all of the perspectives.

As explanatory models drive treatment modalities, multiple modes of understanding will encourage different therapeutic strategies; however, these should converge on the ultimate goal of resolving the experience of sleeplessness. Each model has a different conceptual way of getting there. Just as a patient's insomnia history simultaneously can be viewed with different understandings, various treatment approaches can be seen as incorporating the therapeutic goals of several perspectives concurrently. For instance, developing with a patient a set of instructions regarding evening routines, the timing of sleep opportunities, and general sleep-healthy behaviors can promote the motivated behavior objective of maximizing the homeostatic and circadian sleepiness drive when one is attempting to sleep, counter dimensional vulnerabilities from phase extremes, offer hope and escape from the insomnia victimization seen in the life-story realm, and attempt to cure the hyperarousal syndrome posited in the disease model.

The motivated behavior perspective highlights the sleepiness drive. Therefore, it is especially valuable in identifying situations in which behaviors contribute to undermining the maximum potential of the drive enhancing sleepiness when one is attempting to sleep. Evaluation in this realm must encompass the entire pattern of sleep and sleepiness throughout the 24-hour cycle and consider varying schedules that may encourage one to attempt sleep at circadian phases of arousal. The clinician must have a full appreciation of when the person attempts sleep (including naps) and what happens, of how much sleep the person actually gets, and of any regularity in the timing or circumstances of the reported sleeplessness. Having a patient maintain a sleep log for at least several weeks can be quite helpful in identifying the circadian and homeostatic context of the reported sleeplessness. A graphic sleep log offers a visual representation of the insomnia complaint and may reveal a pattern indicative of an obvious intrinsic or extrinsic behavior problem related to the sleep-wake cycle. This general assessment of the circadian-homeostatic sleepiness drive should represent the foundation of any evaluation of chronic insomnia. Unless identified problems in this fundamental sleep-drive context are addressed, attempts to correct insomnia-promoting influences highlighted by the other perspectives may be fruitless.

Aside from highlighting the factors intrinsically associated with diminished sleepiness, the motivated behavior approach allows a balance analogy to facilitate the consideration of a variety of factors that might contribute to either sleepiness or arousal and therefore to sleep propensity at any particular moment of the day or night. For the time of reported sleeplessness, lists of factors can be made to represent potential problems on the two sides of the balance: those processes decreasing sleepiness or increasing arousal. Specific problems hypothesized as interfering with sleepiness at the desired sleep time can be addressed, often through changes in behavior. Insights from the other perspectives may contribute additional factors to the lists and ultimately should help provide a foundation for the comprehensive case formulation and treatment plan. This process of hypothesis development and testing may be rather fluid—changing over time with new information and feedback from therapeutic experimentation.

The dimensional perspective encourages exploration of longstanding vulnerabilities that might contribute to the development of a person's insomnia experience. People at the extremes of circadian predisposition, the severe early birds and night owls, predictably experience sleeplessness when attempting sleep during otherwise normal schedules. Individuals characterized as having excessive degrees of particular personality features also may be viewed as more vulnerable to sleeplessness. The identified features will influence the approach to treatment, which might include manipulations of circadian rhythm, schedule changes, and perhaps psychotherapeutic and behavioral strategies.

In the evaluation of insomnia, the life-story perspective encourages a search for the cause of insomnia in the remote and recent past and considers the current role of insomnia in the person's life. Insomnia is seen as an understandable reaction to certain situations. In the patient's present life, maladaptive behaviors—routines and habits—may reinforce the insomnia experience. Treatment can focus on changing either the circumstances or how the person responds to them. Since the insomnia represents an ongoing story, an attempt can be made to rescript the narrative and can incorporate hope for improvement with sleep and overall functioning.

The disease perspective appr[...] understanding of insomnia through syndromes, patholo[...] d etiology. Insomnia may be explained as a sympto[...] as a primary disorder with its own presum[...] and cure the underlying problem [...] horough review of any ps[...] edication effects that

[...]nia together promote [...]able and, in some cases, vital [...]eep difficulty. Each is like a lens or [...]on of the same complex view—the patient [...]laint. The product of the initial evaluation of a [...]nia probably will be recognition of various factors th[...] contributing to the sleep disturbance. A formal diagnosis of ins[...]ia may be recorded; however, this will not necessarily capture the variety of influences and nuances of the individual's case, nor will it automatically direct the appropriate treatment strategies. As noted in chapter 1, the development of a valuable, criteria-based nosology of insomnia has been challenging because insomnia is not one, or even 20, separate disorders that can be easily delineated. It is always a complaint, and only sometimes is it a disorder. Therefore, in addition to the administratively necessary diagnosis attribution, a patient's case should be summarized with a more extensive discussion that elucidates the salient features of the clinical situation, as this will be particularly important regarding treatment options. With time, this formulation may evolve with new information and therapeutic feedback.

The Formulation of Insomnia

A logical progression in formulating an insomnia case may begin with the aspects of the sleepiness drive, highlighting any clear problems associated with the circadian and homeostatic processes. The clinician first should

question whether it makes sense that the patient complains of sleeplessness at the time he or she is attempting sleep. Is this insomnia at *this hour*
predictable? Do the patient's behaviors maximize sleep propensity for the
time that he or she wants to be sleeping?

Next, enduring predispositions may be considered. Does this person
have an intrinsic vulnerability for insomnia due to longstanding dimensional features, such as personality characteristics or an extreme position
along the spectrum of early bird to night owl? Is this insomnia at this hour
in *this person* predictable?

Next, the life context of the person complaining of insomnia can be
reviewed to explore situations in his or her past and present that might
contribute to the sleep disturbance and to consider how the insomnia currently affects the person. Are there routines and cognitions that seem to
reinforce chronic insomnia? Is this insomnia at this hour in this person
who is in *this situation* predictable?

Only now should the clinician consider insomnia as a symptom in formulating the patient's case. Short-circuiting the process by immediately
explaining the insomnia as a result of the patient's depressed mood, back
pain, restless legs, or syndrome of conditioned hyperarousal bypasses the
opportunity to assess more fundamental sleep-related vulnerabilities and
to help create a more comprehensive environment conducive to an
improved sleep experience. At this point the clinician should review in
detail medical, psychiatric, and sleep disorders, as well as the effects of
medications and other substances. Is this insomnia at this hour in this person who is in this situation and with *this disorder* predictable?

As in all clinical evaluations, the history is the foundation of the
patient's assessment. Especially in the area of sleep medicine, additional
informants, particularly bed partners and other household members, can
valuably supplement the information provided by the patient. Previous
medical records and laboratory findings also may provide important data.
Questionnaires inquiring about the presence and frequency of particular
sleep-related symptoms can aid in the assessment process. The value of a
graphic sleep log has been emphasized. The information gathered may
then direct further means of evaluation, such as sleep laboratory testing
or clinical consultations. The complexity of many cases of chronic insomnia, including multiple comorbidities, makes collaborative management
essential.

Insomnia Cases

Brief case descriptions, mostly of patients evaluated in the Sleep Disorders Center at Johns Hopkins, have been presented thus far with the intention of illustrating salient features of each of the four perspectives. If, while considering these case descriptions, the reader has contemplated alternative interpretations of the patients' situations, that broader thinking would be entirely consistent with the thrust of this book. These brief case presentations, and certainly the patients seeking help for insomnia in clinical settings, should be examined from multiple perspectives, as is suggested in the examples below.

> *The Disabled Night Owl:* Martha was 52 years old when she came to the Sleep Disorders Center seeking help with her sleep problems, which she blamed for her inability to work. She said that throughout her life she had found it easy to stay up and then sleep late the following day. However, for decades she was able to manage a normal work schedule, and she had been rather successful at her company. Beginning about five years before her visit, she started to experience persistent difficulty falling asleep at night. Generally, it was not until 2:00 to 4:00 A.M. before she could fall asleep. Soon she was sleeping through her 7:30 A.M. alarm. She was able to arrange a later start time at work, but this was only a temporary solution. On days that she was not working, she always would sleep until some time in the afternoon. Increasingly, she missed days at work and eventually she was terminated. At that point she regularly was sleeping from about 5:00 A.M. until at least 2:00 P.M., and she was feeling very discouraged about sleeping her life away. Usually, she felt wide awake throughout the evening and well into the night. She had tried taking hypnotic medications around midnight, but these seemed to have little effect in promoting an earlier sleep onset. Her history included several episodes of major depression and two psychiatric hospitalizations, the first of which had occurred soon after the birth of her son. She had experienced no recurrences during the past 10 years, and she attributed this to her continued use of phenelzine during this period. Her history also included alcohol abuse, but she now had been abstinent for five years. She had been divorced for 12 years and was living alone. At the time of her sleep center evaluation, she reported that, although she was rather frustrated, she felt very motivated to conquer her current problems and return to full-time employment. She had no identified medical disorders, and she

was on no medications, other than the phenelzine. Her physical examination was unremarkable.

The focus of Martha's complaint was a worsening difficulty waking up in the morning due to her uncontrollable sleepiness. She had seen several doctors, and disorders of excessive sleepiness, such as narcolepsy, had been contemplated. However, consideration of her sleepiness drive immediately shows that she was able to attain sufficient sleep, although at a very inconvenient time, and she felt fully alert throughout her waking hours. As she slept later into the daytime, she further reduced the potential for morning light exposure, which could have been helpful in maintaining a somewhat earlier sleep-wake cycle. Unfortunately, her circadian system was promoting sleep mostly during the daytime. Clearly, she experienced a significant vulnerability due to her extreme position along the spectrum of circadian phase predisposition, such that she drifted into the severe night owl pattern.

There were no obvious pervasive personality vulnerabilities associated with Martha's sleep cycle problems. Although she did have episodes of depression, this was not a persistent characteristic and generally was not a major problem for her during the period of worsening daytime sleepiness. From a life-story viewpoint, the sleep problem did cause tremendous life difficulties for her, but these were mostly the result and not a cause. Nevertheless, her eventual circumstances—unemployment—allowed further deterioration to an even later sleep cycle timing. She interpreted the daytime sleepiness as a major challenge that she needed to overcome to get on with her life. The disease model allows a specific diagnosis—delayed sleep phase syndrome. The understanding of her history as consistent with this syndrome offers explanation for the past and suggests treatment approaches to promote an advance in her circadian system. Disease reasoning also raises the question of any possible influence of her history of mood disorder on her recent sleep problems. Certainly, depression could have contributed to her problem by causing social withdrawal and decreased motivation to get out of bed and out of her house. The potential sleep-related effects of her use of the phenelzine cannot be established; however, some individuals do experience excessive daytime sleepiness and disrupted nighttime sleep while taking this medication. Martha was very grateful to the phenelzine for helping to prevent further depressive episodes, and she would not consider a trial without it.

Martha's treatment included education about the disorder, specific guidelines about when she should be in bed, a gradual schedule change over several months, exposure to bright light at her scheduled wake-up time, psychotherapeutic support during a series of follow-up visits, and continued use of her phenelzine. She was pleased with her ability to be awake by 10:00 A.M. every morning, and she was able to return to part-time employment.

The Anxious Early Bird: Yang was a 44-year-old, Chinese woman employed as an educator. Her primary care physician referred her to the Sleep Disorders Center for help with the management of her persistent insomnia symptoms and her increasing distress about her sleep difficulty. She noted that throughout her life she had tended to be an early bird— she felt sleepy most evenings by 8:00 P.M., she usually went to bed and fell asleep quickly at about 10:00 P.M., and she always awoke spontaneously early in the morning, never relying on an alarm clock. For about 20 years she had had occasional sleep difficulty—mostly episodes of awakening excessively early. At the time of her evaluation, she had been experiencing severe early morning awakening persistently for three months. She felt that she slept only about three hours soon after going to bed, and then she remained awake, or in and out of light sleep, for the rest of the night. Recently, her awakenings sometimes were associated with profuse sweating. She was rather frustrated and anxious while awake during the night. During the daytime she felt fatigued and had poor concentration. She worried about how she would sleep the next night. For many years she had occasionally used various herbal, over-the-counter, and prescription agents for sleep, anxiety, and depression. These had included melatonin, Saint John's wort, antihistamines, benzodiazepines, and an assortment of antidepressants. Most recently, she was taking trazodone and alprazolam. Additionally, for two years she had been on Synthroid for hypothyroidism. With hopes of improving her sleep, she was attempting to exercise more in the daytime and early evening, taking a hot bath in the evening, and drinking hot milk at bedtime.

Many potential influences on Yang's insomnia are evident. Generally, she is attempting to sleep at her normal time, and she is not napping during the daytime. Accordingly, she should be experiencing sufficient intrinsic sleepiness at the time she is attempting to sleep. However, she does present a clear history of a circadian phase advance pattern, which increases her vulnerability for awakening in the early morning. Although she has not had treatment by a mental health specialist, over many years she has attempted self-treatment, and primary care physicians have prescribed agents for anxiety and depression. Her anxious predisposition may increase her risk for symptoms of chronic insomnia. Insomnia has been a major theme in her life for many years. However, there were no clear precipitants for the current episode. The disease perspective would raise the question of recurrent major depressive episodes contributing further to her already circadian-predisposed early-morning awakenings. It would be important to confirm that her thyroid medication was not excessively stimulating. Her nighttime sweating episodes raise the question of perimenopausal symptoms with flushing. Finally, the stimulating and/or sedating effects of her various medications and substances would have to be considered. For instance, might bedtime alprazolam, when she does not really need sedation, promote some degree of hyperarousal later during the night as a withdrawal effect?

> *The Napping Pharmacist:* Alfred was an 80-year-old, married, retired pharmacist when he was referred to the Sleep Disorders Center because of his persistent insomnia. He had been satisfied with his sleep until 10 years previously, when he had begun to have problems getting to sleep and staying asleep. He felt that he now never slept for more than one hour consecutively. Recently, he had been going to bed at some point between 11:00 P.M. and 1:00 A.M. Usually, by 2:00 A.M. he would be wide awake, and often he would remain awake for several hours. After finally returning to sleep, he would be awakened around 4:00 A.M. by his dog licking his face when needing to be walked. He then would read the newspaper and eat a small breakfast before returning to bed for another one to two hours of sleep. After that he would take a brisk walk and eat lunch around noon, followed by a nap of 30 to 60 minutes. Overall, he would have interrupted periods of sleep between about midnight and noon and then generally remain awake for the other 12 hours. He had tried various hypnotics over the past five years, but they were of limited help. His wife noted that he snored. His medical history included hypertension, hypothyroidism, and prostatic hypertrophy, and he was taking a diuretic and levothyroxine.

This older man has a multitude of influences potentially undermining his sleep. A consideration of the sleepiness drive reveals predictable sleep difficulty, as he spends half of every day in and out of bed with intermittent sleep. His insufficient nighttime sleep promotes some daytime sleepiness; however, he also is attempting sleep at hours of decreased circadian sleep propensity. There were no clear psychological vulnerabilities, nor was there evidence of an abnormal circadian phase predisposition. His life circumstances, particularly his retirement, had removed much structure from his daily routine. This, in turn, had allowed his sleep-wake schedule to deteriorate, which probably reinforced the problem. There was no evidence of psychiatric illness; however, medical problems and medications may have been promoting nighttime awakenings. His physical examination revealed a weight of 204 pounds (mildly obese for his height) and a narrowed oropharyngeal airway. These, along with the history of snoring, raise the potential arousing influence of sleep-disordered breathing. Finally, assessment of the sleepiness-arousal balance would have to include the dog as yet another awakening influence.

The Devoted Snorer: Jay was 60 years old when he came to the Sleep Disorders Center for evaluation. He had experienced disrupted nighttime sleep since his teens, and over the past few years he had suffered with significant daytime hypersomnolence. He had been living in a religious community and recently had been asked to leave because he regularly fell asleep during morning prayers and was unable to participate in community responsibilities. Typically, he would go to bed about 9:00 P.M. and fall asleep within 30 minutes. He would sleep soundly for about two hours and then have multiple repeated awakenings throughout the rest of the night. He was aware that he snored loudly, and occasionally he awoke with a choking sensation. Often he felt wide awake at times during the night, and sometimes he went to the community chapel to pray. He would get out of bed by 6:30 A.M. to begin his daily activities. During the daytime he was very sleepy, and he would nod off inadvertently several times. Frequently, he fell asleep in the chapel, and he had hit his head on the pew. At times he fell asleep standing up. Nevertheless, he avoided daytime napping because of his concern that the subsequent night would be worse. Although he had denied significant depressive symptoms over the past few years, his psychiatric history did include recurrent major depressive episodes and four psychiatric hospitalizations. His only medication at the time of his evaluation was fluoxetine, which he had been taking for 10 years. His medical history included severe bilateral congenital eye problems, which required multiple surgeries, including a left-sided enucleation. He had only slight light perception on the right side. His physical examination revealed a normal weight but was remarkable for a significantly narrowed oropharyngeal airway and an enlarged uvula. A polysomnographic evaluation demonstrated a severe degree of obstructive sleep apnea.

Clearly, Jay's sleep difficulties had marked ramifications. At least on a theoretical basis, his blindness with minimal light perception may have limited his ability to be entrained to a normal photoperiod, thereby influencing the timing of his intrinsic sleepiness drive. The homeostatic results of his sleep deprivation were profound, with his repeatedly falling asleep during other activities. There did not seem to be a stable circadian timing predisposition or a predictably changing pattern, as demonstrated in the blind free-running case in chapter 3. Nor were there clear personality vulnerabilities. The sleep difficulty did play a major role in his life; however, his life seems to have suffered from the insomnia and hypersomnia rather than the life circumstances contributing to the sleep problem. Psychiatric illness, particularly his recurrent major depressive episodes, probably had influenced his sleep in the past but did not seem to contribute to his current condition. However, with insomnia being a recognized adverse effect of fluoxetine, this medication may have been an influence on his nighttime sleeplessness. Concerning his medical history, the eye pathology was not likely directly contributory, except by way of the possible limitation of circadian entrainment. Finally, he was at significant risk for obstructive sleep apnea because of the loud snoring, airway abnormalities, and severe hypersomnolence. As noted, this sleep disorder diagnosis was confirmed with sleep laboratory testing.

The Bed Hater: Catherine, a 54-year-old, married woman, was seen for evaluation in the Sleep Disorders Center because of persistent insomnia. She had been sleeping fine from about 10:00 P.M. to 6:00 A.M. when she was working full time; however, since she had quit her job seven years previously her nighttime sleep had been severely disrupted. Due to chronic sleep-onset problems, she had given up going to her bed to try to fall asleep. Rather, she would fall asleep on her sofa at some point around midnight after reading or watching television. She noted that she now found her bed too depressing, and she specifically stated, "I hate being in that bed." She would awaken by 3:00 A.M. and feel fully alert. She then would smoke a few cigarettes and after a few hours possibly return to sleep. However, it was not unusual for her to begin her day around 4:00 A.M. with household chores. She estimated that she got between two and five hours of sleep most nights. Her husband had told her that she snored and tended to move in a thrashing manner occasionally while asleep. She described feeling fatigued during the daytime, but she denied sleepiness. In fact, she remarked that she did surprisingly well for "someone who doesn't get much sleep." She said she felt very "keyed up" during the daytime and could not nap even if she tried. She would drink three to four cups of coffee each day, sometimes well into the evening. She often drank several glasses of iced tea during the daytime, and most evenings she would drink one to two glasses of wine. Her psychiatric history included treatment for recurrent major depression over the previous 20 years. In the past she had been prescribed various sedating antidepressants and anxiolytics. For the past year she had been taking bupropion, 300 mg per day. Her weight was in the normal range, and her oropharyngeal airway was narrow.

This patient previously had slept well during usual nighttime sleep hours, but now she typically fell asleep later, woke up earlier, and had prolonged interruptions in between. There do not seem to be primary circadian or homeostatic factors that would directly influence her nighttime sleepiness drive, and there is no evidence of a persistent problem with a circadian timing predisposition. A tally of nighttime sleepiness and arousal balance factors would have to consider the potential stimulation from the excessive caffeine, evening alcohol (hyperarousing withdrawal effects), and nicotine. Catherine does have longstanding anxiety and depressive symptoms; however, it is unclear the degree to which this would represent a personality vulnerability or a manifestation of a primary psychiatric illness. The life story involves a complex narrative of symptoms and her decline from high-functioning employment. Her avoidance of her bed was dramatic; her own story had evolved to a state where her bed had a very negative connotation for her regarding sleep. It is likely that her psychiatric illness had influenced her sleep adversely in the past; however, she recently had been doing well psychiatrically. She may have been experiencing stimulating effects from the bupropion. Her snoring and narrowed oropharyngeal airway raised the possibility of obstructive sleep apnea contributing to her awakenings. There also was a question of periodic limb movements, which could be exacerbated by her previous use of antidepressants. Polysomnographic testing was recommended to evaluate for these primary sleep disorders.

The Early Snorer: Ronald, a 75-year-old, retired police officer, was seen in the Sleep Disorders Center for chronic insomnia, which had begun during World War II. He believed that the stress of his combat experiences was responsible for the onset of his insomnia. The problem had been much worse during the past five years, and he attributed this to his diagnosis of prostate cancer. He felt that both the distress from the diagnosis and his needing to get up to urinate repeatedly during the night were important factors. His typical routine was to retire to his own bedroom at about 6:00 P.M., immediately after his dinner. He would watch television very briefly and soon fall asleep. He said, "TV is my sleeping pill." He thought that he usually was asleep by 7:30 P.M. but would then awaken within 30 minutes. For the rest of the night, he would be up and down and in and out of sleep before finally getting up for the day between 3:00 and 5:00 A.M. Although he slept apart from his wife, she stated that he snored loudly. During the daytime he did not feel sleepy, he never napped, and he had no inadvertent sleep episodes. Although he had drunk alcoholic beverages excessively in the past, he had avoided all alcohol during the previous year. He said that he had had mild symptoms of depression in the past but had never been treated for it. His medical history was remarkable for a stroke in his mid-40s, at which time he retired. He had no residual effects from the stroke and was able to pursue a variety of activities. His weight was 210, down 50 pounds over the previous six months as a result of dieting. His physical examination revealed a significantly narrow oropharyngeal airway.

Ronald's intrinsic sleepiness drive should be adequate during his chosen sleep time; however, there is clear evidence of a marked circadian phase advance pattern. This would account for his ease in falling asleep and his habitual early-morning awakening but not the repeated awakenings throughout his sleep period. There were no obvious enduring psychological vulnerabilities. There are major life-story associations—both in temporal coincidence and in his interpretation. He believed that the recurrent need to urinate was a cause of his awakenings. It might also be argued that his expectation of poor sleep contributed to his sleeplessness. The previous effect of alcohol on his sleep is unclear. Persistent insomnia may continue during long periods of abstinence in people with alcohol dependence. Psychiatric factors also may have been significant in the past, particularly considering his reported combat-related stress and the untreated depressive episodes. The direct effects of the prostate problems and the sense of needing to urinate also are not clear. While awakenings secondary to the need to urinate certainly are common for some individuals, it is not unusual for people to attribute awakenings from other causes (e.g., sleep-disordered breathing) to a need to urinate. Resolution of an underlying problem sometimes can decrease or eliminate the nocturnal urination. Ronald's risk of obstructive sleep apnea is increased due to the snoring, obesity, and airway abnormality.

The Sleepy Security Guard: Lawrence, a 49-year-old, single man, was referred to the Sleep Disorders Center because of his persistent insomnia and increasing daytime sleepiness of about five years duration. He identified the onset of his sleep difficulty as corresponding with the death of his fianc,e. Additionally, he had found his work schedule at that time to be extremely challenging, and he thought that this also interfered with his ability to sleep. Recently, he had been going to bed around midnight and falling asleep within about one hour while watching television. He would sleep with the head of the bed raised considerably so that he could breathe more comfortably and minimize gastroesophageal reflux. He then would awaken repeatedly during the night (about every hour), either with a sense of needing to urinate or from a choking sensation. Finally, he would awaken spontaneously and get up for the day at about 6:00 A.M. He was aware that he snored loudly, as it sometimes awakened him and because others had commented on the noise. Often he felt drowsy during the daytime; however, he avoided napping and he denied inadvertent sleep episodes. He would drink caffeinated beverages throughout the day, often including at least three 20-ounce bottles of soda. He worked full time as a security guard and part time as a driver. He had no psychiatric history. Medical problems included obesity: over the past year his weight had increased 50 pounds, taking him up to 397 pounds on the day of his initial visit. He also had been diagnosed with mild diabetes, hypertension, and gastroesophageal reflux. His only medications were antacids and an oral hypoglycemic. In addition to the obesity, the physical examination revealed a significantly compromised oropharyngeal airway.

Lawrence's evaluation did not demonstrate current sleepiness drive problems secondary to his schedule and his desired sleep hours. Several years previously, when the insomnia had begun, however, he had had a changing work schedule that probably did undermine his ability to achieve adequate sleep. The present and dangerous homeostatic problem was his current excessive sleepiness due to insufficient nighttime sleep. Significant enduring dimensional vulnerabilities, whether circadian phase timing or personality characteristics, were not evident. His own narrative of the sleep history involved the major precipitants of his fiancée's death and the stressful work schedule five years previously. Clearly, now he lived with the expectation of markedly interrupted sleep and impaired daytime functioning because of his sleepiness. Although not included in his own insomnia explanation, except to the extent that he recognized improvement with raising his bed to avoid acid-reflux discomfort, medical and sleep disorders can be seen as major contributory factors promoting his sleep disturbance. He is at very high risk for sleep apnea and dangerous sequelae. His morbid obesity, loud snoring, nighttime choking, abnormal airway, and daytime sleepiness all support a hypothesis of obstructive sleep apnea. The recurrent gastroesophageal reflux promotes even more awakenings. In diabetic patients, inadequate glucose control can promote arousals, especially with precipitous drops in the glucose level during the night. He was immediately scheduled for polysomnographic testing, and the medical issues were addressed collaboratively with his primary care physician.

The Violent Sleeper: Patty, a 42-year-old, married woman, was seen in the Sleep Disorders Center because of her concern about her disrupted nighttime sleep. She noted that she always had tended to be an early bird—waking up early without an alarm clock and restricting her evening activities because of her sleepiness and early bedtime. Typically, she would go to bed and fall asleep by 9:00 P.M. She would awaken spontaneously between 2:00 A.M. and 4:00 A.M. and, knowing that she would not return to sleep, she would then get up for the day. Even when circumstances required a much later bedtime, she still awoke rather early.

Patty was very attentive to her sleep environment. She minimized potentially disturbing light with blackout curtains and an eye mask, and she minimized bothersome noises with earplugs and a bedside fan generating white noise. Generally, she was alert and functioning well during the daytime, but she did feel rather fatigued and sometimes drowsy after the especially early morning awakenings. With hopes of sleeping longer at night, she had occasionally experimented with antihistamines, prescription hypnotics, and sedating antidepressants. Most of these trials resulted in grogginess the following morning. Overall, she felt that her early-morning awakening problem was fairly well controlled.

Her impetus for the sleep evaluation was the disruption of her sleep and further daytime sleepiness due to occasional dramatic episodes of bizarre and sometimes violent behaviors. These episodes always occurred about 30 to 60 minutes after she fell asleep. Typically, she would sit up suddenly and scream loudly. Sometimes she would pound on her husband. He described her as seeming not to be awake, quickly returning to normal sleep, and often not remembering the events. Occasionally, she would awaken fully and describe the episode as extremely terrifying. She had a sense that she was dying and sometimes choking. Occasionally, she would sleepwalk. She worked full time as a nurse. She had no history of psychiatric illness or ongoing medical problems. She had had a hysterectomy four years previously and was taking estradiol. Her weight was normal, and her physical examination was unremarkable.

Patty was concerned about factors that interfered with her ability to achieve sufficient sleep. She was following routines that should have allowed an appropriate sleepiness drive at her desired sleep hours. Her inability to get enough nighttime sleep did promote some homeostatic pressure of daytime sleepiness, depending on the previous night. There was no evidence of personality feature vulnerabilities, but her longstanding early sleep onset and morning awakenings clearly reflected her advanced circadian predisposition. Obviously, this was a powerful determinant of her daily routines. Her markedly advanced phase was an enduring vulnerability that undermined her ability to sustain sleep later during the night and therefore contributed to her insufficient total sleep duration and chronic sleep deprivation. She did not take her ability to sleep for granted. Her own narrative highlighted her great attention to her preparations for optimizing her sleep environment. Although psychiatric and medical problems were not apparent, her parasomnia sleep disorder interrupted her sleep and further contributed to her nighttime sleep insufficiency and the daytime ramifications. Presumably, she had a constitutional vulnerability for the sleep terror events, perhaps in association with high slow-wave sleep activity. The sleep insufficiency promoted by her advanced circadian phase predisposition could have further increased her slow-wave sleep and thereby increased the likelihood of the sleep terrors, which in turn disturbed her sleep even more. A treatment approach addressing the circadian predisposition could allow sleep later in the morning, thereby increasing her total sleep, decreasing the probability of the sleep terrors, and improving her daytime alertness.

The Worrying Executive: Stuart, a 58-year-old, married business executive, was seen in the Sleep Disorders Center. He noted a lifelong tendency toward early awakenings and never needing an alarm clock. He also described himself as a perfectionist and worrier but felt that these characteristics contributed to his success in business. He had experienced several brief insomnia episodes in the past during stressful periods of his life. His current sleep difficulty had persisted for about six months, having begun with his wife's diagnosis and treatment for lung cancer. Although he was able to fall asleep without great difficulty, he now experienced severe early-morning awakening. He would awaken several times during the night and usually have difficulty returning to sleep. Often he had the sense of his mind racing. Some nights he would sleep only two to three hours. During the daytime he felt fatigued and anxious. Previously, napping would have been easy for him, but now he found it impossible. He felt that his work productivity had suffered due to his lack of sleep. After the onset of the insomnia and anxiety, he was prescribed alprazolam during the day and evening, and he found this moderately helpful. Other than the symptoms and treatment noted above, he had no other psychiatric history. His medical history included previous cluster headaches and prostatic hypertrophy. He was of normal weight, and his physical examination was unremarkable.

Stuart was experiencing daytime homeostatic effects of insufficient nighttime sleep; however, they seemed to be offset by the arousing anxiety he experienced. He was not exhibiting behaviors that should have decreased his intrinsic sleepiness drive during his desired nighttime sleep hours. Stuart also has an enduring advanced circadian phase timing predisposition contributing to his insomnia risk during the latter part of the night. It can be argued that his perfectionistic and worrisome nature also represent liabilities that increase his insomnia probability during this stressful period. The life-story context is clear. It makes sense that he is worried and cannot sleep well because of his wife's illness. In the psychiatric realm, a major depressive episode with anxiety and early-morning awakening could be hypothesized although, considering his symptoms, an adjustment disorder would be more likely. He did not have evidence suggestive of other relevant medical or sleep disorders or medication effects.

The Ruminating Secretary: Rita was a 50-year-old, divorced secretary who came to the Sleep Disorders Center because of her worsening insomnia. She reported that she had been having trouble with her sleep for at least 30 years and that she had a tendency to wake up too early, no matter the day of the week or whether she was on vacation. She never used an alarm clock. Intermittently and especially recently, she also had difficulty falling asleep. Although she might feel sleepy earlier, typically she would get in bed around 10:00 P.M., read for about 30 minutes, and then, on a good night, fall asleep quickly. She always then would awaken by 3:00 A.M., at which point she would feel distressed about how she might feel and function the next day and would worry about whether she would be able to return to sleep. Often during the night she would ruminate about plans for the next day that she might have to cancel. If she did return to sleep, she always was awake again for the day by 5:00 A.M. During the daytime she would feel fatigued and sleepy, especially after a bad night. She said that she was unable to nap and had no inadvertent sleep episodes; however, she minimized her driving because of her concerns about her alertness. She drank two cups of coffee in the morning, and she rarely drank alcoholic beverages. Recently, she had seen a psychiatrist, who prescribed a sedating antidepressant, which was moderately helpful in prolonging her nighttime sleep. She did not have evidence of contributory medical or other primary sleep disorders. Her physical examination was unremarkable.

Rita's case is another example of someone who should have an appropriate intrinsic sleepiness drive but who is suffering from a pronounced advanced circadian phase timing predisposition. She probably would get more nighttime sleep and feel better during the daytime if she allowed herself to fall asleep somewhat earlier in the evening, in accord with her own cycle tendency. However, she also has an enduring personality vulnerability increasing her anxiety proclivity, which is directed toward her self-doubt regarding her sleep. The major theme in her insomnia narrative is that she is a defective sleeper and her entire life suffers as a result. The nightly recurrence of her early awakenings and associated frustration, distress, and anxiety can be seen as promoting a conditioned hyperarousal, which can be interpreted in the disease perspective as a syndrome. A primary psychiatric illness also may be contributing to some degree of anxiety and mild depression.

Rita shared a significant advanced circadian timing predisposition with the patients in the previous two examples. In her case, there was a superimposed disease model syndrome of conditioned hyperarousal. If she had not had the advanced circadian vulnerability, she may never have had the insomnia stimulus to worry about her sleep and functioning, and, thus, the conditioned anxiety and hyperarousal may never have evolved. In Stuart's case, superimposed on the patient's advanced sleep timing predisposition was the life-story perspective of worry regarding his wife's illness. Finally, Patty's advanced pattern vulnerability, which limited her total nighttime sleep duration, contributed to her worsened sleep in the context of her parasomnia sleep disorder.

These 10 cases have helped illuminate both the value and the logic of considering explanations derived from the four distinct perspective models. Each one can emphasize important processes and relationships relevant to a patient's insomnia complaint. In some situations, the patient's behavior undermines the sleepiness drive, enduring personal characteristics increase the insomnia risk, life situations stimulate and reinforce the sleep disturbance, and insomnia as a symptom may be integral to a primary disorder. The specific organization presented here is not offered as the ultimate solution for the evaluation of patients complaining of insomnia. Rather, it suggests that a comprehensive evaluation of insomnia must be broad based and must consider influences within these general realms.

Developmental Trends and Insomnia

Although people of all ages experience insomnia at different times for an assortment of reasons, certain broad generalizations are possible. The likelihood of intrinsic and extrinsic factors can be influenced by age. Life events, schedule demands, habits and routines, circadian timing predisposition, biological changes, the risk of various disorders (psychiatric, medical, and sleep), and medication and substance use all generally may have different influences at different life stages. The end result is the epidemiological evidence showing that the complaint of insomnia increases steadily with age.

Newborns do not have an organized circadian system, and thus there is no underlying cycle promoting the timing of sleepiness and sleep. Fortunately, there is the homeostatic drive of sleepiness; however, sleep initially is distributed throughout the day and night. The differentiation of nighttime sleep and daytime wakefulness evolves gradually over a period of many months and even years (considering routine napping). Young children have a relatively high homeostatic sleep need, typically at least 10 hours a day. Insomnia is a rare complaint among children. When it does occur, often explanation is offered in the realm of family relationships, with models from the dimensional and life-story perspectives. Children are at the greatest risk for enuresis and the non–rapid eye movement (NREM) parasomnias (i.e., sleepwalking, sleep terrors) that may disrupt their sleep and that of other household members.

With puberty there commonly is a phase delay in the circadian system, such that there is a greater tendency for teenagers to go to bed later and sleep later the next day. Habits may reinforce the delay, but the biological system allows a strong permissive influence. Often teens simply are not sleepy and are unable to fall asleep at a normal bedtime of 10:00 to 11:00 P.M. The effects typically are more dramatic with the struggle to get out of bed in the morning, when physiologically they may still be in the circadian zone of profound sleepiness. Most teenagers experience this delay to a mild extent, but for some it is severe. When this cycle delay does cause significant problems, it may generate a clinical evaluation. The primary complaint may be insomnia or excessive daytime sleepiness and associated school and work impairment.

Many young adults will continue to experience an increased phase-delay risk. The challenges of work schedules and the demands of family responsibilities further compound the complexity of maximizing the influences of homeostatic and circadian sleepiness at the time allotted for sleeping. Young adulthood also brings new life circumstances and adaptations. Parenthood challenges the ability to achieve sufficient sleep in many ways. A person's own narrative of chronic insomnia may be well established by this time, with a persistent worry about each night's sleep. And, during these years, the use of various substances, such as caffeine and alcohol, can influence the ability to sleep.

In the later adult years, people still may be exposed to significant schedule challenges, particularly due to occupational demands. Some people find that they no longer can sleep sufficiently and function adequately on the shift work schedules they tolerated when younger. Increasingly for those in their 40s, 50s, and 60s, there is greater risk for many psychiatric, medical, and sleep-related processes that may undermine a positive sleep experience. With age, of course, the risk of exposure to medications that potentially can influence sleep will increase. In a general sense, these factors will culminate in the geriatric population, where a constellation of processes increasing the risk of insomnia may be present.

Geriatric Insomnia

Surveys of community-living elders typically show that more than half report difficulty initiating or maintaining sleep or persistent early-morning awakening. Many older individuals say that their sleep now is very light and never reaches the depth they recall experiencing when they were younger. Laboratory studies have documented the tendency for increased arousals and awakenings from sleep, as well as a decrease in slow-wave sleep, in healthy geriatric populations. Daytime fatigue, sleepiness, and napping often accompany the insomnia of elderly persons. Complaints of insomnia are so common among older individuals that some people even regard sleep disturbance as an inevitable consequence of aging. The perspectives approach can help illuminate some of the factors that may contribute to the magnitude of the insomnia problem in the geriatric population.

From the motivated behavior perspective, we can question whether there is a sufficient sleepiness drive to promote rapid sleep onset and to help sleep continue for an adequate duration. Routine napping immediately raises the issue of the homeostatic process. Nighttime insomnia and afternoon napping can evolve into a detrimental cycle. On the other hand, napping can allow some older individuals to feel and function better during their waking hours. No matter what the cause, extended periods in bed throughout the 24-hour cycle can move one toward the "homeostatic breakdown" extreme described in chapter 3. Sleep distributed intermittently during the day and night undermines the sleepiness drive, as significant homeostatic sleep pressure may not be able to build up and there is no reinforcement of a circadian differentiation between day and night. Some older individuals are less able to be exposed regularly or sufficiently to entraining influences, such as bright light, which otherwise might reinforce their circadian timing and amplitude.

Hypotheses regarding age-related intrinsic changes in the sleepiness drive resulting from homeostatic and circadian processes assume neurological pathology and therefore would overlap with disease reasoning. The result could be a fundamental deficit in the degree to which the older brain can accumulate sleep deprivation to promote adequate sleepiness or in the extent to which it can generate the electrical activity associated with deeper sleep. Circadian abnormality could involve an intrinsically blunted amplitude, which, hypothetically, would cause less nighttime sleepiness and daytime arousal. Thus far, the evidence for these arguments has been equivocal.

Enduring vulnerabilities emphasized with the dimensional perspective may prominently influence geriatric insomnia. Certainly, personality characteristics still may be contributory in promoting chronic insomnia, especially as more sleep interruptions from other causes may be present as precipitants. However, almost universal among elderly persons is the shift in the circadian phase to an earlier timing. This factor may be the sole cause of early-morning awakening or the experience of light and interrupted sleep during the latter part of the night. Alternatively, this phase advance may increase the likelihood of arousals and awakenings from other causes during this part of the night. Since the phase-advance tendency occurs with aging in most individuals, those who began as early birds, though not necessarily suffering from insomnia when younger, are at the greatest risk for the further advance that can cause significant insomnia symptoms. As noted in chapter 4, this phase-advance tendency is often an unrecognized factor in the insomnia of older individuals.

Major life changes often accompany aging, and these may contribute to geriatric insomnia from the life-story perspective. Obvious are the losses of spouses and other family members and friends. Older individuals may have to move from the setting of decades of comfortable sleep to a new residence or even an institutional setting. One's own narrative changes with the recognition of physical and functional limitations, and this may promote anxiety and demoralization that can impair sleep. The insomnia interpretation an older individual assumes may be that sleep always is bad in elderly persons, and therefore they do not seek help for the problem.

While circumstances can play a role in causing insomnia, the opposite also may be true. Sleep disturbance may bring about changes in life circumstances. Disruption of the sleep-wake cycle may be a key factor leading to nursing home placement. Family members caring for an older relative with dementia at home may no longer be able to manage the situation when no one in the house is able to get adequate sleep at nighttime.

The disease perspective highlights many potential factors in the etiology of insomnia. Clearly, the geriatric population overall is at the greatest risk for many medical, psychiatric, and primary sleep disorders that can promote insomnia as a symptom. These may include acute and chronic disorders, especially those associated with pain and discomfort. Cardiovascular, pulmonary, neurodegenerative, and prostatic disorders are notable examples. Mood disorders, particularly major depression, as well as anxiety and adjustment disorders also may be prominent in this population. Sleep-disordered breathing and the related restless legs syndrome and periodic limb movements may be present but not immediately apparent. The parasomnia rapid eye movement (REM) behavior disorder, which can disrupt sleep rather dramatically, is most common among elderly individuals.

Elderly persons are more likely to be on multiple medications and also may be more vulnerable to adverse effects secondary to age-related pharmacokinetic and pharmacodynamic changes. Excessive nighttime stimulation (e.g., some antidepressants and antihypertensives) and sleep disruption (e.g., diuretics) and daytime sedating effects all can undermine the sleep-arousal balance that normally supports a healthy sleep-wake cycle.

Disease model reasoning also encourages theoretical advances, empirical data collection, and new collaborative research endeavors. At least in the theoretical realm, this perspective can stimulate etiological questions regarding the relatively high prevalence of insomnia in older individuals. Perhaps age-related neurodegenerative processes directly contribute to impairment in sleep-generating mechanisms. Conceivably, a future test might indicate the presence of a particular primary insomnia etiological process.

Women and Insomnia

Large surveys of the general population typically show that the female sex represents an added risk for the insomnia complaint, particularly for the age groups beginning in the mid-40s. Of course, the sleep disturbances that women experience mostly are those processes that also may affect men and are those that have been elaborated throughout this book. However, unique aspects of female physiology and life cycle may further heighten the potential for disturbed sleep. The menstrual cycle, pregnancy stages and the postpartum period, and the transition into menopause and the subsequent postmenopausal phase all may be associated with brief or extended episodes of sleeplessness (Walsleben and Baron-Faust, 2000).

Many women experience a predictable deterioration in their ability to sleep satisfactorily during premenstrual days or during the first few days of the menstrual period. Often there is an associated complaint of discomfort, such as from bloating or cramping; however, in many other cases insomnia is the primary symptom. A mood disturbance also may accompany the menstrual-related insomnia. In rare cases women predictably experience a profound and debilitating hypersomnolence before or during the menstrual period.

Insomnia is a very common complaint during pregnancy. Some sleep difficulty is almost universal among women during the last trimester. Physical discomfort, frequent bathroom visits, gastroesophageal reflux, and fetal movements all can interfere with sleep. Also with pregnancy is an increased risk of sleep-disordered breathing and restless legs syndrome. Insomnia, excessive sleepiness, and fatigue may become problems even during the first trimester.

Disturbed sleep may continue during the postpartum period, in part for presumed physiological reasons, but the insomnia is compounded further by nighttime feedings and general concerns about the newborn baby. Many women report that suddenly with motherhood they never slept deeply again—sensing a perpetual attentiveness for their children's needs. With significant postpartum insomnia, the clinician should always consider the possibility of a depressive disorder.

Insomnia is one of the hallmarks of the perimenopausal period and subsequent menopause. Many women complain of a gradual decline in their ability to sleep deeply enough or long enough, beginning at some point ranging from their early 40s to early 50s. Superimposed on this decline may be dramatic autonomic arousals of hot flashes, which may occur several times during a single night and continue episodically for years.

In the disease model, hormones are the easy explanation for much of the sleep difficulties unique to women. Research does suggest that sleepiness can be influenced by the levels, fluctuations, and balances among estrogen, progesterone, testosterone, luteinizing hormone (LH), and follicle-stimulating hormone (FSH). The normal late-luteal phase drop in progesterone and estrogen may contribute to premenstrual insomnia through a decrease in sleepiness. Analogous processes may help explain the insomnia of the postpartum period and during menopause. However, the understanding of hormonal influence on brain function and regulation of the sleep-wake cycle remains incomplete. Although these influences probably are of critical importance, issues of individual vulnerability and life circumstances surely affect a woman's proclivity for insomnia. Pregnancy may be one woman's supreme joy and another's nightmare. Menopause may be welcomed as a relief from menstruation or viewed primarily as the beginning of life's final stage.

Treatment Modalities and the Perspectives

The treatment of patients complaining of insomnia should be individualized and should flow from the formulation of their cases. The underlying argument of this book has been that a multitude of processes may influence the potential for insomnia and that many of these factors may be operating simultaneously. Therefore, various treatment approaches may be indicated for any particular person. Of course, this is not unusual in clinical practice. For instance, hypertension may be addressed with a dietary program (e.g., salt restriction), weight loss, exercise, and assorted medications with different pharmacodynamic actions. The identification of multiple insomnia influences, however, does not necessarily require disparate and uncoordinated treatment programs. Often therapeutic strategies can incorporate goals crossing perspective boundaries.

All of us experience brief episodes of insomnia at some time in our lives. Usually, there are clear situational precipitants. Typically, the stimulus resolves or we adapt to the situation, so these brief insomnia episodes often do not come to clinical attention. However, people do sometimes seek help for their sleep while in the midst of some crisis. Perhaps an immediate cause can be addressed. Additionally, psychotherapeutic support and possibly the temporary use of a short-acting hypnotic may be beneficial. Sometimes this early treatment can help prevent longer-term sleep difficulty.

What is the ideal clinical setting for the evaluation and treatment of chronic insomnia? This, too, is dependent on the patient and the clinical circumstances. Ideally, the evaluator will be able to offer a comprehensive consideration of the broad range of processes (e.g., behaviors, enduring vulnerabilities, life circumstances, and disorders) potentially contributing to the patient's sleep disturbance. Treatment options then may include such strategies as schedule modifications, behavior changes, the exposure to or avoidance of bright light at particular hours, substance restrictions, behavioral therapy and psychotherapeutic techniques, hypnotic medications, and direct attention to other contributory disorders (which may warrant further testing and treatments). The global treatment plan for insomnia may have the patient work with various practitioners to accomplish the therapeutic objectives. The overall insomnia evaluation and treatment may be coordinated and conducted by a single clinician, with considerable individualization in modalities and timing. Alternatively, chronic insomnia may be approached successfully with a highly structured generalized treatment program, such as that espoused by Charles Morin (1993). His insomnia program incorporates weekly group therapy sessions that emphasize particular themes each week. There is a strong cognitive-behavioral foundation, with a broad range of sleep-healthy recommendations.

Patient education always should be at the foundation of the clinical management of chronic insomnia. Patients should understand how their behaviors, vulnerabilities, situations, and disorders can affect their sleep and contribute to their insomnia. Patient insight into these processes will help motivate compliance with treatment recommendations, which otherwise might be met with more resistance. Knowledge about basic sleep-regulation mechanisms may help patients face new circumstances with better solutions. Furthermore, explanation is reassuring, which inherently may be therapeutic.

Time and patience also are important ingredients in the management of chronic insomnia. Sometimes patients come in for help, demanding an instant solution to the sleep problems with which they have suffered for years. Rapid improvement in sleep sometimes is possible, but more commonly recovery is a longer-term process. The treatment plan may include immediate steps (e.g., evening coffee cessation, use of hypnotics) and approaches requiring longer periods for effective results (e.g., psychotherapy, use of antidepressants). Monitoring the outcome of different therapeutic manipulations can enhance the patient-clinician partnership as the successes or failures of various strategies are explored. The hypotheses of the formulation of a patient's insomnia complaints may be confirmed, revised, or discarded. Ongoing clinical care allows continued feedback and modification of the treatment plan, as well as continued support and encouragement.

Just as each of the perspectives of insomnia illuminates different aspects of a patient's case and highlights factors that might influence the risk for that person's sleep difficulty, the perspectives also suggest different, though complementary, treatment strategies. Often an identified problem directly leads to a treatment objective and plan. General therapeutic directions associated with the motivated behavior, dimensional, life-story, and disease perspectives are considered in the following four sections.

The Motivated Behavior Perspective and Treatment

The motivated behavior perspective helps elucidate factors that may interfere with an appropriate degree of sleepiness at the desired time for sleep.

An appreciation of the homeostatic process in sleep regulation reveals the importance of the daily schedule in fostering satisfying sleep. Sufficient time (e.g., 16 hours) between sleep episodes normally enhances sleepiness; therefore, intervening sleep episodes, as with napping and other extended periods in bed with intermittent sleep, may be identified as potential problems. Further impetus for schedule regularization comes with an understanding of the critical influence of the circadian cycle on sleep. Since the circadian rhythm incorporates an intrinsic fluctuation in sleepiness, the ability to initiate and sustain sleep will be maximized when one schedules sleep regularly and in accord with the circadian system. Because of the normal entrainment with the photoperiod, in humans sleepiness is generally the greatest during the nighttime.

Many patients with chronic insomnia will benefit from establishing a sensible schedule that allows the same period of approximately eight hours reserved for the opportunity of sleep each night. A reliably completed graphic sleep log readily will show deviations from the recommended schedule and will give a subjective representation of overall sleep efficiency and particular times of sleep difficulty. Such a schedule for ideal sleep hours requires no competing activities that would interfere with the sleep opportunity; however, whether the insomnia patient should remain in bed awaiting sleep for the entire period is a matter to consider with other perspectives. The motivated behavior approach is useful in suggesting the physiological time period that should be most conducive to satisfying sleep.

The balance analogy of processes potentially contributing to sleepiness or arousal at desired sleep times can have a practical application. The time period associated with insomnia can be considered with regard to the individual factors that might cause insufficient sleepiness, on the one hand, and excessive arousal, on the other. As discussed in chapter 3, insufficient sleepiness might result from too much sleep over the previous day or from attempting to sleep at a time not in synchronization with the circadian sleepiness drive. Many processes may be viewed as arousing and thereby possibly contributing to the insomnia. Lists of these factors can be helpful in developing a treatment plan, particularly where possible behavioral changes are highlighted. Some arousing influences can be addressed relatively easily (e.g., napping, caffeine). Adverse work schedules, chronic pain, and distress due to financial problems are much less easily addressed. Nevertheless, elaborating all of these potential negative influences on sleep contributes to the explanatory framework of the case.

Widely published lists of recommendations for sleep hygiene typically include some items that represent arousing influences that can undermine sleep. For instance, the avoidance of caffeine, alcohol, and late-evening strenuous exercise often are included. The potential direct stimulation of features in one's sleep environment also may be on these sleep hygiene lists. Commonly, a cool, dark, and quiet bedroom is suggested as ideal. People do tend to experience somewhat more consolidated sleep in a slightly cool room, as long as they are sufficiently covered and not uncomfortable. Relative darkness during the sleep hours should minimize possible stimulating effects. Absolute darkness may be unsafe, if one needs to get up during the night. However, turning on bright lights during nighttime bathroom visits can have a direct stimulating effect and possibly a negative circadian influence, as well. Accordingly, very dim nightlights, especially in bathrooms, may be useful. The amount of light one should seek or avoid before or after the sleep period may depend on issues of circadian predisposition emphasized in the discussion on the dimensional perspective.

Absolute silence may not represent the ideal sleep environment for many people. Especially when attempting to fall asleep, some people find that, in the complete absence of sound, they listen very intently for any noise. They may dwell on whether they are actually hearing something. Certainly, intrusive sounds, such as barking dogs, nearby traffic, and that from television and radio should be minimized. Many people sleep better with constant white noise, which not only can help block out disturbing outside noises but also seems to have a soothing influence that can enhance sleep. This background white noise can be achieved with a specific noise-generating device or rather easily with a bedside fan.

The treatment issues underscored with the motivated behavior perspective mostly relate to maximizing the opportunity for sleep. This means creating an internal and external environment that is as conducive as possible to the onset and maintenance of sleep. The individual's daily schedule and behaviors should maximize sleepiness when sleep is attempted, and the surroundings should minimize interruptions of sleep. This general sleep milieu can be seen as the foundation of chronic insomnia treatment. Resolution of the sleep problem may be achieved entirely in this realm. Treatment approaches associated with causes of insomnia emphasized in the other perspectives still should benefit from attention to these fundamental sleep influences.

The Dimensional Perspective and Treatment

In this book, dimensional influences have been examined in terms of the enduring vulnerabilities increasing the risk of insomnia that may exist in the realms of personality features and of sleep-related characteristics, particularly the circadian phase predisposition. One or more components of a patient's treatment plan can be directed toward reducing the risk resulting from any identified predisposition.

Personality characteristics seen as contributing to chronic insomnia are summarized with the construct of internalization, wherein people habitually do not overtly express their emotions. These individuals tend to be ruminative, pessimistic, and self-deprecating. When attempting to sleep, they experience excessive emotional arousal, which leads to physiological activation and insomnia. Several strategies have been proposed to counter this maladaptive pattern, which seems to promote symptoms of chronic insomnia. Since these persons deal poorly with stress, stress reduction, whenever possible, should be helpful. More important, psychotherapy can help them change how they respond to stressful situations and learn how to better express their emotions, particularly anger. Relaxation techniques may help alleviate the arousal and activation that occurs at bedtime. Therefore, among the options considered for treating chronic insomnia should be a plan that incorporates these psychotherapeutic, stress reduction, and relaxation objectives.

The advanced and delayed circadian phase predispositions may profoundly influence the risk for insomnia, especially for early-morning awakening and difficulty falling asleep, respectively. The resulting sleep disturbances may be lifelong, at least from the teen years onward, or may relate to the major developmental trend of the phase delay among teenagers and young adults and the phase advance among elderly individuals. Imparting an understanding of the persistent influence of the circadian system on insomnia symptoms is the first step in treatment. The individual may be able to obtain a sufficient amount and quality of sleep with a shift in the planned sleep time. Other therapeutic strategies may help shift the circadian system enough to allow a more rapid sleep onset in the phase-delayed patients and more sustained sleep in the phase-advanced insomnia sufferers.

Among living organisms, light, typically by way of the natural photoperiod, is a primary entraining factor for the circadian system. In humans, light in the hours before the nighttime sleep period can have a phase-delaying effect on the timing of the circadian clock, and light in the hours after the nighttime sleep period can have a phase-advancing effect. These effects are greater with brighter light and, consistent with an experimental phase-response curve, with light at a time closer to the sleep period. The absence of bright light may allow the opposite effects to occur. As the circadian system shifts, so does the associated timing of the sleepiness rhythm.

In phase-advanced individuals, an increase in evening exposure to bright light and a decrease in exposure to morning light, particularly around dawn, may promote a delay in the circadian sleepiness that will be beneficial in treating the early-morning awakenings and very light sleep that these patients experience. Although household lights in the evening may be satisfactory to promote a mild phase-delay effect, the proper use of a therapeutic bright light box at a regular time most evenings may be necessary for a satisfactory response. The exact time and duration of the exposure to bright light may need to be determined by experimentation with the patient. Thirty minutes every evening at 8:30 P.M. will be therapeutic for some phase-advanced patients, while others may require at least one hour. Morning light can be minimized with dark or blackout curtains, and soft eyeshades also can be worn. Patients often argue that there is no need to avoid morning light, since they are awakening while it is still dark. The key issue is not the direct stimulating and potentially awakening effect of the light but rather the phase-advancing influence of the light in these individuals who already are too phase advanced. Concerted attention to these adjustments in light exposure have great potential in alleviating disrupting early-morning awakening, especially in elderly persons who have drifted into this pattern over the previous few years.

The phase-delayed individuals, who are predisposed to stay up late and sleep well into the following daytime, may benefit from the opposite guidelines. That is, they should minimize exposure to bright light in the evening and maximize exposure to light after the sleep period. Many of them have been doing just the opposite, which presumably has had a permissive effect in worsening the phase delay that already was a constitutional vulnerability. This night owl population tends to be somewhat recalcitrant to treatment, as many have difficulty maintaining an established schedule. The significantly phase-delayed insomniac individuals often have very irregular schedules—getting up early when necessary and sleeping late whenever possible. Even when they do make some progress, their sleep-wake cycles tend to drift later when circumstances do not require an earlier awakening. In this way they lose some ground that previously had been achieved in shifting their cycles earlier.

A practical treatment approach for the phase-delayed patients should include the establishment of a reasonable time at which they can arise for the day. Choosing an earlier time that will not be followed will be fruitless. An excessively early rising time risks promoting a further detrimental phase delay by falling on the delay portion of the phase-response curve. Patients may be exposed to bright light at the scheduled awakening time, presumably during the morning daytime hours or in rather severe cases even in the afternoon. While a therapeutic light box may be valuable in the treatment of these patients, the daytime awakening allows the use of sunlight as the source of light. Again, the exact duration and timing may need to be determined empirically, and gradually the scheduled awakening and light exposure can be shifted earlier. As suggested in chapter 4, it is important for the patients to give themselves the opportunity to fall asleep gradually earlier than they have been accustomed.

In the future, other phase-shifting strategies may be available to help the patients at these two circadian extremes of the phase-advanced and phase-delayed patterns. Although evidence for the use of melatonin as a bedtime hypnotic has been equivocal, there is compelling experimental evidence that it functions as a modulator of the timing of the circadian system. Alfred Lewy and Robert Sack (1997) demonstrated that low-dose melatonin can be beneficial for both of these groups of patients with circadian rhythm disorder. They gave multiple doses of small amounts of melatonin in the afternoon and evening to phase-delayed patients, and they gave morning doses to phase-advanced patients. In both situations there was generally an improvement in the symptoms. The melatonin is thought to have a phase-response curve relative to shifts of the circadian system that essentially is the opposite of the light exposure curve. Presumably, the bright light and melatonin can act in concert when given at opposite times.

The Life-Story Perspective and Treatment

The life-story perspective explains insomnia through the narrative logic of history. Patients offer stories about why they cannot sleep, and clinicians elaborate their own interpretations for the causes of the symptoms. These causes of insomnia are found in the past and present circumstances of the lives of insomnia sufferers. Broad examples include distressing situations acutely promoting sleep difficulty and ongoing psychological reinforcement in the environment where sleeplessness is experienced, thereby leading to chronic insomnia. In this realm of the narrative explanation of insomnia, interpretation and treatment are interwoven. As noted in chapter 5, the major explanatory models of insomnia incorporate intrinsic treatment strategies. In fact, these theoretical orientations generally are described with labels that actually refer to the treatment: sleep restriction, stimulus control, and cognitive-behavioral therapy. The essential features of each of these approaches to insomnia treatment are described in chapter 5. While each strategy can be applied in a pure form, most commonly the insights and techniques of these orientations are combined in the treatment plan for insomnia patients.

The potential value of the psychotherapeutic process is emphasized in the life-story perspective. With acute or chronic insomnia, there may be recent or current situational factors that can be addressed directly. Patients may be able to change circumstances or how they respond to them, and they also may be supported through difficult times. The treatment of all insomnia sufferers should respect the narratives that they bring forth, even when the stories are not fully in accord with clinicians' interpretations and formulations. The effective treatment of insomnia, particularly in chronic cases, often will involve a reshaping of these narratives. Of course, hope has an important narrative role. The clinician-patient relationship can help promote in insomnia sufferers a transition from victimhood to agent of change. A central feature of the cognitive-behavioral approach is the correction of cognitive distortions—the maladaptive beliefs that seem to contribute to ongoing distress and sleeplessness. Often there is an expectation of the inability to sleep and an excessive fear of the consequences. For all of these reasons, the clinician-patient relationship is an important component of the therapeutic process.

Both specific and general treatment recommendations emerge from insomnia explanation in the life-story perspective. The purported detrimental influences of excessive time in bed and conditioned hyperarousal in promoting symptoms of chronic insomnia are within this domain. The circumstances are seen as sustaining the sleeplessness. Since the evening routines, bedtime, bedroom, and the bed itself can be viewed as stimulating and reinforcing insomnia-related anxiety, it may be argued that patients should avoid the bedroom when not sleepy and avoid the bed, within reason, when not asleep. "To bed or not to bed?"—that is the question for many insomniac persons who wonder whether they are better off resting in bed or getting up to do something else when they cannot sleep. Ultimately, the recommendation depends on the formulation of the case. The presence of anxiety and frustration while sleepless in bed does suggest the potential value of a treatment plan incorporating aspects of the stimulus control and sleep restriction approaches.

Most generally, in the life-story perspective, treatment means identifying the key features in patients' lives that are viewed as causing and sustaining their insomnia. The role of their own insomnia stories also must be considered. Therapeutic interventions then can serve to eliminate, where possible, processes interpreted as promoting and sustaining the insomnia symptoms. This may involve changing routines, beliefs, and expectations. The outcome will incorporate a new narrative.

The Disease Perspective and Treatment

Insomnia is explained in the disease model in terms of syndromes, pathology, and etiology. Accordingly, insomnia is understood as a symptom of another disorder or as an intrinsic feature of its own disorder. The solution to the insomnia problem simply may involve the identification, treatment, and optimization of any medical, psychiatric, and other underlying sleep disorders that might contribute to the insomnia symptoms. However, since the symptoms of the other disorders may not be resolved rapidly or perhaps not at all, then other measures may be warranted. Chronic insomnia patients who are regarded as having an intrinsic insomnia disorder, such as those diagnosed with primary insomnia or psychophysiological insomnia, generally are treated by sleep medicine specialists in a rather broad manner—combining therapeutic features highlighted in all four of the perspectives described in this book. Often this will incorporate sleep-related education, schedule advice, substance precautions, behavioral recommendations, some degree of supportive or insight-oriented therapy, and possibly hypnotic medications, exposure to or avoidance of bright light, and assorted relaxation strategies.

The penultimate goal in the disease model is the discovery of the etiology responsible for pathology causing the symptoms of an identified syndrome. The ultimate goal is a cure. Hypotheses of possible intrinsic insomnia diseases are presented in chapter 6. It has been argued that sleep problems may result from pathology in circadian physiology, the autonomic nervous system, brain electrophysiology, and psychological processes, among others. An etiology of genetic abnormality can be proposed. Although there may be promise in these proposals, presently there is no firm recognition of a broken bodily part that can be repaired to improve sleep. We hope the future will bring new insights and creative solutions.

Symptomatic relief has been sought in the use of substances with actual or supposed sedating properties. Physicians have prescribed various types of medications to help patients sleep better. Advances have led to the current generation of hypnotic medications (e.g., zolpidem, zaleplon) that generally promote a rapid sleep onset but have a duration of action sufficiently short not to cause sedation the following day. The relatively short half-lives prevent accumulation from occurring. Withdrawal effects have been shown to be minimal or absent. For these reasons, physicians and patients have been more accepting of the use of medications in the management of acute and chronic insomnia.

There is no established cure for insomnia, for the simple reason that insomnia itself is not an established disease. However, insomnia always is treatable in some manner. An assortment of syndromes include insomnia as a symptom, and these can be approached by using the wide variety of specific and general therapeutic modalities now available. The disease perspective encourages the recognition of particular symptom constellations so that explanation can be pursued and treatment effectiveness can be predicted. Significant progress has been made in recognizing different insomnia syndromes and therapeutics, but many questions remain unanswered and solutions are yet to be discovered.

Summary

The motivated behavior, dimensional, life-story, and disease perspectives each illuminate aspects of the sources of insomnia. The sleepiness drive and its balance with arousal are emphasized in the motivated behavior paradigm. Enduring personal vulnerabilities that may influence the ability to sleep satisfactorily are seen with the dimensional perspective. How the circumstances and narrative in one's history result in insomnia are elucidated with the life-story approach. Insomnia as a symptom of various syndromes and how it may represent its own disorder are explored with the disease model. Any or all of these domains of explanation may simultaneously contribute to the understanding of an insomnia patient's case.

The evaluation of individual patients with insomnia, as well as an appreciation of the global processes contributing to the experience of sleeplessness, benefits from a broad approach that considers multiple influences. There is no single explanation and no single solution for everyone. People complain of insomnia for many different reasons, and this diversity and complexity should be reflected in the formulation of their cases. The consideration of these multiple perspectives helps demonstrate key developmental and life-stage issues that may be relevant to the risk of the insomnia experience. Potential physiological, psychological, and social changes may be important for different age groups and genders.

The treatment of insomnia may involve approaches associated with the various explanations that are derived from the different perspectives. Explaining insomnia from different viewpoints will help the clinician seeking to understand cases more fully and manage patients more effectively. The more influences that are appreciated, the better we can target complementary treatment strategies. Therapeutic modalities might include schedule regularization, strategic exposure to light, behavioral changes, medications, and psychotherapy, among many others. The integration of these approaches into a patient's treatment plan ensures the best possible outcome.

Appendix

Sleep Medicine Resources

Comprehensive Textbooks of Sleep Medicine

Principles and Practice of Sleep Medicine, third edition. Edited by Meir H. Kryger, Thomas Roth, and William C. Dement. Philadelphia: W. B. Saunders Company, 2000.

Sleep Disorders Medicine: Basic Science, Technical Considerations, and Clinical Aspects, second edition. Edited by Sudhansu Chokroverty. Philadelphia: Butterworth Heinemann, 1999.

Journals

Behavioral Sleep Medicine (Lawrence Erlbaum Associates)

Journal of Sleep Research (Blackwell Science and the European Sleep Research Society)

Sleep (American Academy of Sleep Medicine and the Sleep Research Society)
www.journalsleep.org.

Sleep Medicine (Elsevier Science)
www.elsevier.com/locate/sleep

Sleep Medicine Reviews (Elsevier Science)
www.elsevier.com/locate/smrv

Sleep Research Online
www.sro.com

Organizations and Foundations

American Academy of Sleep Medicine
www.aasmnet.org
Sleep Research Society
www.sleepresearchsociety.org
Society for Light Treatment and Biological Rhythms
www.sltbr.org

179

National Sleep Foundation
www.sleepfoundation.org

Governmental Organizations

National Center for Sleep Disorders Research
www.nhlbi.nih.gov/about/ncsdr

Sleep Websites

Sleep Home Pages
www.sleephomepages.org
Sleep Medicine Home Page
www.users.cloud9.net/~thorpy

References

American Medical Association. 1996. *International Classification of Diseases, 9th Revision, Clinical Modification* (ICD-9-CM). Salt Lake City: Medicode.

American Psychiatric Association. 1994. *Diagnostic and Statistical Manual of Mental Disorders*, 4th ed. Washington, D.C.: American Psychiatric Association Press.

Ancoli-Israel, S., and Kripke, D. F. 1989. Now I lay me down to sleep: The problem of sleep fragmentation in elderly and demented residents of nursing homes. *Bulletin of Clinical Neurosciences* 54:127–32.

Ancoli-Israel, S., and Roth, T. 1999. Characteristics of insomnia in the United States: Results of the 1991 National Sleep Foundation Survey. *Sleep* 22(suppl 2):S347–53.

Balkin, T., Thorne, D., Sing, H., Thomas, M., Redmond, D., Wesensten, N., Williams, J., Hall, S., and Belenky, G. 2000. Effects of Sleep Schedules on Commercial Motor Vehicle Driver Performance. U.S. Department of Transportation, Federal Motor Carrier Safety Administration, Report DOT-MC-00133, MAY.

Beullens, J. 1999. Determinants of insomnia in relatively healthy elderly: A literature review. *Tijdschrift voor Gerontologie en Geriatrie* 30:31–38.

Bixler, E. O., Kales, A., Soldatos, C. R., Kales, J. D., and Healey, S. 1979. Prevalence of sleep disorders in the Los Angeles metropolitan area. *American Journal of Psychiatry* 136:1257–62.

Bliwise, D. L. 1993. Sleep in normal aging and dementia. *Sleep* 16:40–81.

Bliwise, D. L., Friedman, L., Nekich, J. C., et al. 1995. Prediction of outcome in behaviorally based insomnia treatments. *Journal of Behavior Therapy and Experimental Psychiatry* 26:17–23.

Bonnet, M. H., and Arand, D. L. 1997. Hyperarousal and insomnia. *Sleep Medicine Reviews* 1(2):97–108.

Bootzin, R. R., and Nicassio, P. M. 1978. Behavioral treatments for insomnia. *Progress in Behavior Modification* 6:1–45.

Bootzin, R. R., and Perlis, M. L. 1992. Nonpharmacologic treatments of insomnia. *Journal of Clinical Psychiatry* 53, no. 6 (suppl):37–41.

Breslau, N., Roth, T., Rosenthal, L., and Andreski, P. 1996. Sleep disturbance and psychiatric disorders: A longitudinal epidemiological study of young adults. *Biological Psychiatry* 39:411–18.

181

Broughton, R. 1994. Important underemphasized aspects of sleep onset. In: *Sleep Onset: Normal and Abnormal Processes*, edited by Ogilvie, R. D., and Harsh, J. R., 19–35. Washington, D.C.: American Psychological Association.

Campbell, S. S., Murphy, P. J., van den Heuvel, C. J., Roberts, M. L., and Stauble, T. N. 1999. Etiology and treatment of intrinsic circadian rhythm sleep disorders. *Sleep Medicine Reviews* 3:179–200.

Carskadon, M. A., and Rechtschaffen, A. 2000. Monitoring and staging human sleep. In: *Principles and Practice of Sleep Medicine*, 3d ed., edited by Kryger, M. H., Roth, T., and Dement, W. C., 1197–1215. Philadelphia: W. B. Saunders.

Carskadon, M., Dement, W., Mitler, M., et al. 1976. Self report versus sleep laboratory findings in 122 drug free subjects with the complaint of chronic insomnia. *American Journal of Psychiatry* 133:1382–88.

Chang, P., Ford, D., Mead, L., et al. 1997. Insomnia in young men and subsequent depression. *American Journal of Epidemiology* 146:105–14.

Czeisler, C. A., and Khalsa, S. B. 2000. The human circadian timing system and sleep-wake regulation. In: *Principles and Practice of Sleep Medicine*, 3d ed., edited by Kryger, M. H., Roth, T., and Dement, W. C., 353–75. Philadelphia: W. B. Saunders.

Czeisler, C. A., and Wright, K. P. 1999. Influence of light on circadian rhythmicity in humans. In: *Regulation of Sleep and Circadian Rhythms*, edited by Turek, F. W., and Zee, P. C., 149–80. New York: Marcel Dekker.

Czeisler, C. A., Duffy, J. F., Shanahan, T. L., Brown, E. N., Mitchell, J. F., Rimmer, D. W., Ronda, J. M., Silva, E. J., Allan, J. S., Emens, J. S., Dijk, D. J., and Kronauer, R. E. 1999. Stability, precision, and near 24–hour period of the human circadian pacemaker. *Science* 284:2177–81.

Diagnostic Classification Steering Committee (Thorpy, M. J., chair). 1990. *International Classification of Sleep Disorders: Diagnostic and Coding Manual*. Rochester, Minn.: American Sleep Disorders Association.

Dijk, D. J., and Edgar, D. M. 1999. Circadian and homeostatic control of wakefulness and sleep. In: *Regulation of Sleep and Circadian Rhythms*, edited by Turek, F. W., and Zee, P. C., 111–47. New York: Marcel Dekker.

Dinges, D. F., and Powell, J. W. 1985. Microcomputer analyses of performance on a portable, simple visual RT task during sustained operations. *Behavior Research Methods, Instruments, and Computers* 17:652–55.

Dorsey, C., and Bootzin, R. R. 1997. Subjective and psychophysiologic insomnia: An examination of tendency and personality. *Biological Psychiatry* 41:209–16.

Edinger, J. D., Wohlgemuth, W. K., Radtke, R. A., Marsh, G. R., and Quillian, R. E. 2001. Cognitive behavioral therapy for treatment of chronic primary insomnia: A randomized controlled trial. *JAMA* 285:1856–64.

Everson, C. A. 1995. Functional consequences of sustained sleep deprivation in the rat. *Behavior Brain Research* 69:43–54.

Ford, D. E., and Kamerow, D. B. 1989. Epidemiologic study of sleep disturbances and psychiatric disorders: An opportunity for prevention? *JAMA* 262: 1479–84.

Giles, D. E., Kupfer, D. J., Rush, A. J., and Roffwarg, H. P. 1998. Controlled comparison of electrophysiological sleep in families of probands with unipolar depression. *American Journal of Psychiatry* 155:192–99.

Gillin, J. C., and Byerley, W. F. 1990. The diagnosis and management of insomnia. *New England Journal of Medicine* 322:239–48.

Gulevich, G., Dement, W., and Johnson, L. 1966. Psychiatric and EEG observations on a case of prolonged (264 hours) wakefulness. *Archives of General Psychiatry* 15:29–35.

Hauri, P., Linde, S., and Westbrook, P. 1996. *No More Sleepless Nights.* New York: John Wiley & Sons.

Healey, E. S., Kales, A., Monroe, L. J., Bixler, E. O., Chamberlin, K., and Soldatos, C. 1981. Onset of insomnia: Role of life-stress events. *Psychosomatic Medicine* 43:439–51.

Hoddes, E., Zarcone, V., Smyth, H., et al. 1973. Quantification of sleepiness: A new approach. *Psychophysiology* 10:431–36.

Horne, J., and Ostberg, O. 1976. A self-assessment questionnaire to determine morningness-eveningness in human circadian rhythms. *International Journal of Chronobiology* 4:97–110.

Johns, M. W. 1991. A new method for measuring daytime sleepiness: The Epworth Sleepiness Scale. *Sleep* 14:540–45.

Johnson, L. C., and Spinweber, C. L. 1983. Good and poor sleepers differ in Navy performance. *Military Medicine* 248:727–31.

Jones, C. R., Campbell, S. S., Zone, S. E., Cooper, F., DeSano, A., Murphy, P. J., Jones, B., Czajkowski, L., and Ptacek, L. J. 1999. Familial advanced sleep-phase syndrome: A short-period circadian rhythm variant in humans. *Nature Medicine* 5:1062–65.

Kales, A., and Kales, J. D. 1984. *Evaluation and Treatment of Insomnia.* New York: Oxford University Press.

Kalogjera-Sackellares, D., and Cartwright, R. D. 1997. Comparison of MMPI profiles in medically and psychologically based insomnia. *Psychiatry Research* 70:49–56.

Katz, D. A., and McHorney, C. A. 1998. Clinical correlates of insomnia in patients with chronic insomnia. *Archives of Internal Medicine* 158:1099–1107.

Krueger, J. M., and Fang, J. 2000. Host defense. In: *Principles and Practice of Sleep Medicine,* 3d ed., edited by Kryger, M. H., Roth, T., and Dement, W. C., 255–65. Philadelphia: W. B. Saunders.

Lavie, P. 1989. To nap, perchance to sleep: Ultradian aspects of napping. In: *Sleep and Alertness: Chronobiological, Behavioral, and Medical Aspects of Napping,* edited by Dinges, D. F., and Broughton, R. J., 99–120. New York: Raven Press.

Lewy, A. J., and Sack, R. L. 1997. Exogenous melatonin's phase-shifting effects on the endogenous melatonin profile in sighted humans: A brief review and critique of the literature. *Journal of Biological Rhythms* 12:588–94.

Loomis, A. L., Harvey, E. N., and Hobart, G. A. 1936. Electrical potentials of the human brain. *Journal of Experimental Psychology* 19:249–79.

Lundh, L. G., and Broman, J. E. 2000. Insomnia as an interaction between sleep-interfering and sleep-interpreting processes. *Journal of Psychosomatic Research* 49:299–310.

McCarley, R. W. 1982. REM sleep and depression: Common neurobiological control mechanisms. *American Journal of Psychiatry* 139:565–70.

McHugh, P. R., and Slavney, P. 1998. *The Perspectives of Psychiatry,* 2d ed. Baltimore: Johns Hopkins University Press.

Mignot, E. 2000. Pathophysiology of narcolepsy. In: *Principles and Practice of Sleep Medicine,* 3d ed., edited by Kryger, M. H., Roth, T., and Dement, W. C., 663–75. Philadelphia: W. B. Saunders.

———. 2001. A commentary on the neurobiology of the hypocretin/orexin system. *Neuropsychopharmacology* 25:S5–13.

Mitler, M. M., Gujavarty, K. S., and Browman, C. P. 1982. Maintenance of wakefulness test: A polysomnographic technique for evaluating treatment efficacy in patients with excessive somnolence. *Electroencephalgraphy and Clinical Neurophysiology* 53:658–61.

Moldofsky, H. 1994. Immune-neuroendocrine-thermal mechanisms and the sleep-wake cycle. In: *Sleep Onset: Normal and Abnormal Processes,* edited by Olgilvie, R. D., and Harsh, J. R., 37–50. Washington, D.C.: American Psychological Association.

———. 1995. Sleep and the immune system. *International Journal of Immunopharmacology* 17:649–54.

Moldofsky, H., Scarisbrick, P., England, R., and Smyth, E. 1975. Musculoskeletal symptoms and non-REM sleep disturbance in patients with "fibrositis syndrome" and healthy subjects. *Psychosomatic Medicine* 37:341–51.

Monroe, L. J. 1967. Psychological and physiological differences between good and poor sleepers. *Journal of Abnormal Psychology* 72:255–64.

Morin, C. M. 1993. *Insomnia: Psychological Assessment and Management.* New York: Guilford Press.

Morin, C. M., Colecchi, C., Stone, J., Sood, R., and Brink, D. 1999. Behavioral and pharmacological therapies for late-life insomnia: A randomized controlled trial. *JAMA* 281:991–99.

Niedermeyer, E., Jankel, W. R., and Uematsu, S. 1986. Falling asleep: Observations and thoughts. *American Journal of EEG Technology* 26:165–75.

Owens, J. F., and Matthews, K. A. 1998. Sleep disturbance in healthy middle-aged women. *Maturitas* 30:40–50.

Perlis, M. L., Giles, D. E., Buysse, D. J., Thase, M. E., Tu, X., and Kupfer, D. J. 1997. Which depressive symptoms are related to which sleep electroencephalographic variables? *Biological Psychiatry* 15:904–13.

Perlis, M. L., Smith, M. T., Andrews, P. J., Orff, H., and Giles, D. E. 2001. Beta/gamma EEG activity in patients with primary and secondary insomnia and good sleeper controls. *Sleep* 24:110–17.

Punjabi, N. M., Welch, D., and Strohl, K. 2000. Sleep disorders in regional sleep centers: A national cooperative study. *Sleep* 23:471–80.

Rechtschaffen A. 1994. Sleep onset: Conceptual issues. In: *Sleep Onset: Normal and Abnormal Processes*, edited by Ogilvie, R. D., and Harsh, J. R., 3–17. Washington, D.C.: American Psychological Association.

Rechtschaffen, A., and Kales, A., eds. 1968. *A Manual of Standardized Terminology: Techniques and Scoring System for Sleep Stages of Human Subjects*. Los Angeles: UCLA Brain Information Service/Brain Research Institute.

Rosen, R. C., Rosekind, M., Rosevear, C., Cole, W. E., and Dement, W. C. 1993. Physician education in sleep and sleep disorders: A national survey of U.S. medical schools. *Sleep* 16:249–54.

Sack, R. L., Brandes, R. W., Kendall, A. R., and Lewy, A. J. 2000. Entrainment of free-running circadian rhythms by melatonin in blind people. *New England Journal of Medicine* 343:1070–77.

Santamaria, J., and Chiappa, K. H. 1987. The EEG of drowsiness in normal adults. *Journal of Clinical Neurophysiology* 4:327–82.

Siegel, J. M. 2000. Brainstem mechanisms generating REM sleep. In: *Principles and Practice of Sleep Medicine*, 3d ed., edited by Kryger, M. H., Roth, T., and Dement, W. C., 112–33. Philadelphia: W. B. Saunders.

Simon, G. E., and VonKorff, M. 1997. Prevalence, burden, and treatment of insomnia in primary care. *American Journal of Psychiatry* 154:1417–23.

Spiegel, K., Leproult, R., and Van Cauter, E. 1999. Impact of sleep debt on metabolic and endocrine function. *Lancet* 354:1435–39.

Spielman, A. J., Saskin, P., and Thorpy, M. J. 1987. Treatment of chronic insomnia by restriction of time in bed. *Sleep* 10:45–56.

Stepanski, E. J. 2000. Behavioral therapy for insomnia. In: *Principles and Practice of Sleep Medicine*, 3d ed., edited by Kryger, M. H., Roth, T., and Dement, W. C., 647–56. Philadelphia: W. B. Saunders.

Stoller, M. K. 1994. Economic effects of insomnia. *Clinical Therapeutics* 16:873–97.

Thorpy, M. 1992. The clinical use of the Multiple Sleep Latency Test: The Standards of Practice Committee of the American Sleep Disorders Association. *Sleep* 15:268–76.

Tobler, I. 2000. Phylogeny of sleep regulation. In: *Principles and Practice of Sleep Medicine*, 3d ed., edited by Kryger, M. H., Roth, T., and Dement, W. C., 72–81. Philadelphia: W. B. Saunders.

van Cauter, E. 2000. Physiology. In: *Principles and Practice of Sleep Medicine*, 3d ed., edited by Kryger, M. H., Roth, T., and Dement, W. C., 266–78. Philadelphia: W. B. Saunders.

van Kammen, D. P., van Kammen, W. M., Peters, J., et al. 1986. CSF MHPG: Sleep and psychosis in schizophrenia. *Clinical Neuropharmacology* 9(suppl 4):575–77.

Vgontzas, A. N., Bixler, E. O., Lin, H. M., Prolo, P., Mastorakos, G., Vela-Bueno, A., Kales, A., and Chrousos, G. P. 2001. Chronic insomnia is associated with nyctohemeral activation of the hypothalamic-pituitary-adrenal axis: Clinical implications. *Journal of Clinical Endocrinology and Metabolism* 86:3787–94.

Vincent, N. K., and Walker, J. R. 2000. Perfectionism and chronic insomnia. *Journal of Psychosomatic Research* 49:349–54.

Walsh, J. K., and Engelhardt, C. L. 1999. The direct economic costs of insomnia in the United States for 1995. *Sleep* 22(suppl 2):S386–93.

Walsleben, J., and Baron-Faust, R. 2000. *A Woman's Guide to Sleep.* New York: Crown Publishers.

Wehr, T. A. 1992. In short photoperiods, human sleep is biphasic. *Journal of Sleep Research* 1:103–7.

Wehr, T. A., Goodwin, F. K., Wirz-Justice, A., Breitmaier, J., and Craig, C. 1982. Forty-eight-hour sleep-wake cycles in manic-depressive illness. *Archives of General Psychiatry* 39:559–65.

Wehr, T. A., Moul, D. E., Barbato, G., et al. 1993. Conservation of photoperiod-responsive mechanisms in humans. *American Journal of Physiology* 265: R846–57.

Wisor, J. P., and Takahashi, J. S. 1999. Molecular genetic approaches to the identity and function of circadian clock genes. In: *Regulation of Sleep and Circadian Rhythms,* edited by Turek, F. W., and Zee, P. C., 369–95. New York: Marcel Dekker.

Worthman, C. M., and Melby, M. 2002. Toward a comparative developmental ecology of human sleep. In: *Adolescent Sleep Patterns: Biological, Social, and Psychological Influences,* edited by Carskadon, M. A., 69–117. New York: Cambridge University Press.

Yoss, R. E., Moyer, N. J., and Hollenhorst, R. W. 1970. Pupil size and spontaneous papillary waves associated with alertness, drowsiness, and sleep. *Neurology* 20:545–54.

Zammit, G. K., Weiner, J., Damato, N., Sillup, G. P., and McMillan, C. A. 1999. Quality of life in people with insomnia. *Sleep* 22(suppl 2):S379–85.

Zepelin, H. 2000. Mammalian sleep. In: *Principles and Practice of Sleep Medicine,* 3d ed., edited by Kryger, M. H., Roth, T., and Dement, W. C., 82–92. Philadelphia: W. B. Saunders.

Zlomanczuk, P., and Schwartz, W. J. 1999. Cellular and molecular mechanisms of circadian rhythms in mammals. In: *Regulation of Sleep and Circadian Rhythms,* edited by Turek, F. W., and Zee, P. C., 309–42. New York: Marcel Dekker.

Zorick, F. J., and Walsh, J. K. 2000. Evaluation and management of insomnia: An overview. In: *Principles and Practice of Sleep Medicine,* 3d ed., edited by Kryger, M. H., Roth, T., and Dement, W. C., 615–23. Philadelphia: W. B. Saunders.

Index